8-13-74

MANIPULATION

MANIPULATION

Dangers and Benefits of Brain Research

Erwin Lausch

Translated from the German by
OLIVER COBURN

1974

The Viking Press New York

I would like to express my thanks to
Dr. Andrew Mayes for his help
and advice on the translation.
O.C.

1817264

CONTENTS

INTRODUCTION   7

1 Investigations on Isolated Live Brains   13

2 Brain Research Till Modern Times   26

3 The Split Brain   37

4 The Evolution of the Brain   51

5 Charting the Cortex   59

6 Surgery for the Psyche?   82

7 Feelings to Order   94

8 The Brain's Interior   101

9 Electrical Manipulation   114

10 Chemical Manipulation   122

11 Psychoactive Drugs   129

12 The Nerve Cells 152

13 The Transmitting of Electrical Signals 161

14 The Chemistry of Psychology 177

15 Secret Order in the Jungle 184

16 The Brain as Data-Processor 201

17 Dark-Room of Nightmares 212

18 Sleep and Dreams 225

19 Manipulating Memory 244

20 Apollo Programme for Brain Research 264

BIBLIOGRAPHY 269

INDEX 277

MANIPULATION

INTRODUCTION

Man's Schizophrenic Adventure

The human brain investigates itself

Try to imagine a firm with an office staff of ten to fifteen thousand millions—more than there are people on the earth today—and that they are all telephoning at the same time. Each department has a switchboard which allows connections to be established in fractions of a second with the outside world or other departments.

Such a monster office is no nightmare of the future; each of us already has one in his own head. The London anatomist J. Z. Young used the office analogy to give at least some concrete idea of the human brain's incredible complexity: every one of the ten to fifteen thousand million nerve cells in the brain is connected to thousands of other nerve cells by a vast network through which streams of communications are constantly flowing in all directions.

The human brain, however, is not really at all like a simple telephone switchboard. Research workers are trying in many laboratories to find out what it is and how it actually functions. Experts in many disciplines are collaborating: anatomists and physiologists, psychologists and neurologists, ethologists,

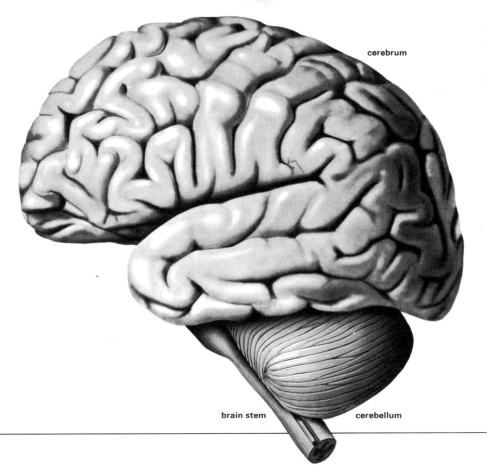

The greatest challenge for science: the human brain.

biochemists, physicists, mathematicians, cyberneticists, computer engineers . . .

As Walter Rosenblith of Massachusetts Institute of Technology put it, exaggerating slightly in his exuberance:

'All the sciences which man's brain has created can now contribute to our understanding of that very brain.'

The two handfuls of greyish, gelatinous matter in our skull present today the greatest challenge for science.

No other subject of research seems to have such a special

fascination. Understandably; for the human brain is by far the most complex organ which nature has produced. It is the organ which makes each human being into an individual, giving that individual his or her personality with all its strengths and weaknesses. It is, in fact, the part of our body which contains the secret of humanity—whatever one may understand by that phrase.

The 'switchboard' in our head, outwardly so unimpressive, controls and regulates all muscular movements; hundreds of muscular systems are co-ordinated in the human body, which is capable of the marvellous sensitivity and precision shown, for instance, by a prima ballerina or a concert pianist. At every moment vast masses of sense impressions come together in our brain, linked to a very subtle code. They are sorted into 'important' or 'unimportant', converted to impulses for movements or reflections, quickly forgotten again or preserved for a long time as memories. Here is stored the experience of a lifetime, in a storeroom with a capacity which seems incredible in view of its tiny physical size. And here, in the human brain, is the most mysterious thing of all: consciousness, whereby we can recognise the universe around us and also the existence of our own brains.

'Brain research', said the Australian neurophysiologist Sir John Eccles, who received the Nobel Prize for Medicine in 1963, 'is the elemental problem with which man finds himself confronted'—and he amplified the statement in these terms:

'Ever since the realization that he was a thinking being, man has been trying to understand essentially what he is. This is a very much bigger problem even than trying to discover how the universe began. The point is that but for man's brain no other problem would exist. But for man's brain the whole drama of the cosmos would be played out before empty stalls; nothing would be known to exist, because no observation would be possible; and a better understanding of the brain is likely to lead man to a richer comprehension both of himself and of the world he lives in.'

In recent years new research techniques have given great impetus to brain research. The scientist is drawn more and more to the most exciting adventure of the human mind, the search for itself. For the first decades of this century human imagination was specially fascinated by problems of the material environment. During the 'fifties molecular biologists began to be more talked about than the exponents of other branches of science. Now brain research has moved into the centre of interest.

Scientists have already succeeded in gaining deep insights into the structure and functioning of the brain. Only a beginning, admittedly; but already much of what earlier generations believed to be within a 'spiritual' realm permanently inaccessible to science has been traced back to quite normal physical and chemical laws.

To find out more about the laws which control human behaviour would be of far-reaching importance. Knowledge of the causes of damaging or anti-social ways of behaviour could lead to new forms of therapy. The conflicts under which man suffers are as futile as they are destructive, from everyday quarrels to mutual slaughter between nations; they could perhaps be avoided, if we only knew more about our brain. Could not battles and wars, brutality and violence, be banished to a museum-piece of history, only preserved for the amazement of posterity as a barbaric practice of our unhappy past? A beautiful vision—why should it not come true?

Might it not be possible one day, through new discoveries in brain research, to make brains capable of a higher level of performance? Might not the capacity of memory be more intelligently used, the effectiveness of learning improved, mental decline in old age be delayed? There are already good prospects today of being able to influence the connections between the brain cells in such a way that greater intelligence results. In the future, however, the priority will be not so much to increase still further the capacity of 'elite' intellects; the urgent problem will be to create the best possible conditions of development for the brains of a large part of mankind which today are condemned to be more or less stunted.

Yet obviously there are also incalculable dangers which may arise from the results of brain research. For if scientists can discover down to the smallest details the laws which control human behaviour, these discoveries will put them in the position of having people under their control.

It has been said half-seriously that a man whose brain was appropriately processed soon after birth would be the cheapest robot. Sir John Eccles is very deeply alarmed by the thought that 'brain research may reveal techniques by which people could be made to be efficient members of a totalitarian society: never rebelling but doing exactly what they're told'. Such a result of brain research he considers 'more dangerous than the atomic bomb'.

Work has already started on such techniques for brain manipulation. Electrical stimuli and chemical influences on the brain can produce actions motivated by no external circumstances and also feelings for which there is no organic cause.

But regardless of whether these effects, and the discoveries which follow from them, will in fact lead to abuse, very serious consequences arise. For what are terms like 'personality' and 'character' still worth if it proves that essential human traits can be manipulated by relatively simple operations? What is left of responsibility and conscience, law and morality, the obstinate belief in guilt and innocence, if all kinds of anti-social behaviour are the result of disorders and defects in particular brain mechanisms? Who could then still believe in a soul, let alone an immortal one, or in a God such as the churches proclaim?

'If love and hate, confidence and fear, go back to chemical shifts in the brain,' reflected the science fiction writer Theo Löbsack, 'if they are controllable independently of external experiences, if they can be "turned on" or "switched off" at will, if you can introduce happiness or pain into a man like a pill or can impose them by an electrical stimulus in his brain, what is left of the divinity which is supposed to reveal "the realm of transcendental experience"? God is then driven out of that ivory tower. We live then in a spiritual world which has become diabolically intelligible, which no longer needs God to explain even our morality.'

All these are important reasons for keeping a careful eye on brain research, its methods, results and the consequences which arise from them.

I

Investigations on Isolated Live Brains

The operation had already lasted five hours, but the most difficult part was still to come.

On the operating table lay a young rhesus monkey deeply anaesthetised. He was mercifully spared, at least for the time being, any awareness of what was happening to him. Robert J. White, neurosurgeon at the Western Reserve University in Cleveland, Ohio, had set himself the task of isolating the monkey's brain, completely separating it from the rest of the body, and then examining it—examining it live, that was the problem.

For no other organ in the body perishes so quickly as the brain if there is failure in the blood supply. It needs a fifth of the whole amount of oxygen which the blood carries from the lungs into the body. If the blood supply to the brain is interrupted, the functions of life are extinguished after only a few minutes. In contrast to the heart, attempts at resuscitation are futile.

So even a minor piece of clumsiness while operating could have wrecked the ambitious project. But White had sensitively and patiently worked his way to the crucial stage of the operation. He had severed the spinal cord in the region of the animal's neck, inserted a small T-shaped tube in each of the two cephalic veins, and (as he laconically wrote afterwards in a scientific report) removed in succession 'all the anatomical structures surrounding the brain'. The tubes were then closed. Later the blood would flow through them from the heart-lung machine into the brain.

A brief pause heavy with tension—then everything went very fast. White first tied off the spinal arteries, which contribute only one-fifth to the brain's blood supply, and cut through them below the tie. Now and also afterwards the brain could do without them, if the machine functioned smoothly. Spinal cord and spine were also cut through. Then he tied the cephalic arteries under the inserted T-tube. He opened the connections to the heart-lung machine and severed the cephalic arteries below the ties.

He had now completely severed the brain from the body with which that morning it was still linked in an apparently inalienable unity. The body lay lifeless on the operating table, unnoticed, until an assistant eventually carried out the headless corpse. But the brain lived.

It needed oxygen and energy-giving dextrose from the blood which the machine supplied to it, and it discharged carbon dioxide into the blood. But the main thing was: it worked. That the nerve cells were active was shown by the electroencephalograph (EEG): the jagged lines registered by this machine proved that the brain's functions were intact.

What dreams may come?

It was in 1963 that White first succeeded in this spectacular isolation of a live brain. Since then he has peeled over a hundred brains of rhesus monkeys from their skulls and severed them from their bodies. He has kept them alive for hours, sometimes for days. He has also severed dogs' brains and transplanted them into other dogs. Experiments with isolated brains have long been made in other places besides Cleveland.

In September 1963 White published in *Science*, the American scientific journal with by far the widest circulation, an account of his neurosurgical *tour de force*. Almost at once there was a storm of protest. The question under debate was whether he had overstepped a border which scientists too ought to respect. The arguments on this point have continued till the present day.

I myself, writing now about the isolated brain, am prey to the same medley of conflicting emotions and ideas which flooded my mind when I first read about White's experiment. While I admire the boldness, skill and determination with which he went about it, it also fills me with anxiety and makes me shudder. It is a tricky problem for our human brain, so thirsty for knowledge, to decide what ought and what ought not to be done to other brains, including those of animals. (The whole question of experiments on animals is, of course, a thorny and complex one, which I have no space to discuss in this book.)

Perhaps the most disturbing thing is that we do not know what goes on in an isolated brain; when it wakes from the anaesthetic, is it in any sense aware of the grotesque situation into which the operator has brought it? What does such a solitary brain think of? Is it tormented by fears, does it want to escape? Is it filled with rage at its impotence or sunk in resignation? 'What dreams may come to a disembodied brain,' asked a writer in the British magazine *New Scientist*, 'and what pain, that the mute organ is unable to express?'

We do not know. The brain on the laboratory table might also have quite different feelings. Perhaps it feels joy to be free for good from its ordinary work. Perhaps it feels an amazed exhilaration that it can now for once consider only itself.

'I suppose', said Lee Wolin, experimental psychologist on

White's team, 'that waking, he [the monkey] would feel like an individual subjected to complete paralysis, because when a man is paralysed, he is aware of the senses' absence. Yes, I assume that this monkey knows the absence of the flesh. But with no physical pain, because all the nerves have been cut off. Psychological suffering, I don't know. I have no idea if he would feel happy or unhappy or lonely.'

We have no instrument so far which can give information about this. The graph of brain current registered on EEGs can offer various conclusions regarding healthy and sick brains. But scientists have not yet read off feelings and thoughts from the jagged lines.

Anyhow, White and his colleagues succeeded in gaining contact with isolated brains. Through a probe, which produced minute electrical currents, he stimulated the stumps of the nerves for seeing and hearing. In the intact organism these nerves lead to quite definite areas of the cerebral cortex, and they pass on to these areas what the eyes and ears register. They do not, however, transmit light or sound waves to the cerebral cortex, but electrical signals, into which the perceptions of the sense organs have immediately been transformed. It is only these electrical signals, after they have been processed in the cerebral cortex, which enable us to experience the world of colour and sound we know.

White's isolated brains no longer possessed eyes and ears, so they could no longer react to light and sound waves. But the electrical signals entering the nerve stumps were immediately transmitted into the brain. Measurements at the cerebral cortex showed that the signals arrived. Very probably the solitary brains 'saw' and 'heard' something— without eyes and ears.

That isolated brains react also to normal sense perceptions was shown by A. J. Blomquist and D. D. Gilboe, two scientists in the neurosurgical department at the University Clinic in Madison, Wisconsin, who severed dogs' brains from their bodies and connected them to a heart-lung machine. But the isolated brains were left two possibilities of contact with the outside world: an ear, and a small piece of nose with the nerves which led from there into the brain. Whether stimuli from the outside world arrived 'correctly' was to be shown by electrodes positioned at the places on the cerebral cortex where the brain normally processed them. The experimenters gently touched the remains of the nose with an electrically driven apparatus which vibrated fast, and the recording from the first electrode promptly showed a strong deviation: the part of the brain responsible for sense stimuli from the nose area had registered the touch stimulus. Normally, of course, the brain would not have confined itself to registering the stimulus; it would have told the muscles, withdraw the head at once!

Blomquist and Gilboe made a loud clicking come from a loudspeaker set up about a yard from the dog's intact ear. They immediately saw the reactions on the EEG machine with which a second electrode placed on the cortex was connected. The jagged line registered by the machine shot up to form a huge indentation. So the brain had perceived accurately.

There is impressive evidence, then, that the isolated brain does actually function. But while for all our knowledge it may suffer terrible fears and torments, should such experiments not be abandoned? The question is clearly justified, the answer extremely difficult and complex.

For White and other brain researchers do not, of course, plan their drastic operations in an overweening sense of human omnipotence; they are not merely concerned in doing whatever looks technically possible, nor are they motivated by pure scientific curiosity. Their essential interest is to be able in the future to help patients who are at present beyond their help or who could be more fully helped. For that they must know more about the brain.

The isolated brains offered the possibility for the first time of making exact examinations of certain processes of metabolism in the brain. There is no other way of establishing so precisely what enters the brain with the bloodstream and what quantities of what substances the blood discharges again. Researchers can study on the exposed brain what the central organ of the organism needs for nourishment besides oxygen and dextrose, and what chemicals it produces which are normally carried away into the body. There is a completely unprecedented chance to follow up, for instance, the effects on the brain cells which can be produced by drugs, changes of temperature, infections, etc. According to White:

'The direction of research marked out by the existence of such preparations will in future put us in the position of being able to analyse exactly the biochemical and neurophysiological functions which take place in the brain and which may be considered the physical basis of specialised psychic functions like memory, consciousness and intelligence. . . . For the neurosurgeon the possibility is also of great importance that with this method he can study more exactly the mechanisms which after surgical operations so often lead to brain oedema (the collection of fluid into the brain), to brain failure and so finally to the patient's death.'

Experiments in which White and other brain researchers 'froze' isolated brains cut off from all blood supply, proved particularly illuminating as regards possible benefits for patients. At normal bodily temperature a brain dies irrevocably, if the blood supply is interrupted longer than a few minutes. But a brain cooled down just above freezing-point, White discovered, would survive several hours without blood supply.

The brain's electrical activity ceases; but the brain itself is only in suspended animation. When at the end of the experiment he had blood warmed to body temperature flow through the brain, the electrical activity started up strongly again, directly the temperature of the brain rose above 30°C (86°F).

The results of such experiments encouraged White to carry out operations which only seemed conceivable if the blood supply to the patient's brain could be temporarily interrupted. After his experiences with frozen, isolated brains, he dared to freeze the brains of patients needing operations—where the brain remained excluded from the circulation of blood for up to half an hour.

Even more astonishing results were achieved by three Japanese scientists, I. Suda, K. Kito and C. Adachi, at the Physiology Department in the University of Kobe. They froze live cats' brains, and kept them in the deep freeze for months—at −20°C (−4°F). The brains' electrical activity had already ceased far above freezing-point. But when they carefully thawed out the petrified brains, and a heart-lung machine pumped in fresh, warm cats' blood, it started again. The EEG registered lines which showed no signs of any brain damage. One brain which could later be restored to life from its petrified state spent 203 days in the deep freeze.

However, for it to survive its stay there, the Japanese scientists found, a special preparation was needed. Before they freed the live brain from the anaesthetised cat, they replaced its warm blood by a sodium solution cooled to 10°C (50°F), to which they had added dextran, a synthetic substitute for blood plasma.

While the blood substitute was pulsing through the body, they severed the brain from the body and attached it to a heart-lung machine. Then they gradually added to the sodium solution fifteen per cent glycerine, which had proved an effective antifreeze with other live tissue. Finally they put the brain into a plastic container filled with the same fluid consisting of sodium solution, dextran and glycerine, and put the whole thing in the deep freeze. For resuscitation they first let the brain slowly thaw out, and replaced the glycerine fluid first by sodium solution, then by warm blood.

The significance of these Japanese experiments lies not only in the proof that the brain, master organ of the body, considered so delicate, possesses under certain conditions an almost incredible resistance to cold. An equally exciting result is that it is evidently possible to exchange the blood completely for a substitute fluid—which casts doubt on the widespread doctrine that nerve cells are specially liable to damage from lack of oxygen.

This doctrine rests on medical experience that, of all organs, the brain reacts most sensitively to an interruption of the blood supply, and that only a few minutes after such an interruption it is irreparably damaged and perishes. In his experiments White, too, took account of this apparently irrefutable fact. But the Japanese researchers replaced the blood with a fluid which could not transmit any oxygen to the nerve cells (as it does not contain any). Before the refrigeration, sodium solution alone was pulsing through the cat's brain for over two hours. Even allowing for the fact that the solution was cool and the tissue cooled by it had a relatively small need for oxygen, nerve cells could not be all that sensitive to the lack of oxygen if they survived this test without damage.

The researchers also reached the conclusion that the cause of the brain damage constantly observed, instead of being extreme sensitivity to lack of oxygen, was a very marked vulnerability in the fine blood vessels in the brain. Even after a brief interruption of the blood stream the venules (small veins) could no longer open and so caused a continuous loss of oxygen. Obviously it may be very important medically to know the real cause of the brain's sensitivity to circulatory troubles.

Brain transplants

Understandably, the experiments with isolated brains

immediately aroused speculations as to whether they would one day lead to brain transplants. If a man's brain was incurably damaged, for instance by a car crash, might the body not be equipped with the healthy brain of another man who has been carried off, say, by a heart attack? If live brains can be kept fresh for months in the deep freeze, why not establish brain banks which would keep a suitable brain ready for all requirements?

Brains have in fact been connected already with a foreign organism. As early as the 'fifties the Soviet surgeon Vladimir Petrovich Demichov in Moscow carried out a series of experiments in transplanting brains, with results which made headlines all over the world as 'Dogs with Two Heads'. But actually it was the whole front half of a small dog which was transplanted, brain, head, neck and front paws. Demichov sewed it into a big dog's neck. The transplanted head, after coming out of its anaesthesia, could smell and see, eat and bark. The big dog found the unwonted burden in its neck uncomfortable, and tried to shake it off. This caused pain to the small dog-head. It resisted and bit its carrier in the ear.

Demichov's dog-head transplants, which lived for up to twenty-nine days, were ingenious if creepy experiments, which showed great surgical skill. But they contributed little to transplant research. Speculations about real brain transplants were only possible after White in Cleveland had isolated the brains of rhesus monkeys. For these brains, severed from their bodies, he did more than supply them blood through the heart-lung machine. He often selected a 'live blood-pump'. He connected the solitary brain with the circulation of an anaesthetised rhesus monkey; the monkey's heart easily managed the extra task. A 'transplantation', White wrote, had thus taken place from one live animal to another.

The quotation marks are his. Clearly he realised himself that the expression 'transplantation' was rather too bold for an experimental arrangement whereby one monkey had for a period merely supplied another monkey's brain with blood. In fact, he described an experiment he carried out in 1965 as 'the first successful brain transplantation'. In this experiment, which he repeated several times, he severed a dog's brain from its body, in the same sort of way as he had done before with a monkey's brain. It was much harder with a dog for anatomical reasons, and it took him eight to nine hours; but it had the advantage that dogs cost much less than monkeys. In another dog's neck he prepared a pocket of skin which was to take the isolated brain.

The brain was attached to the receiver dog's cephalic artery and neck vein. After he had lined it with electrodes and equipped it with devices which later allowed him to follow the temperature, blood pressure and composition of the blood, he sewed up the skin pocket. He continued such experiments for up to three days. The transplanted brains functioned splendidly right to the end—as the measuring instruments showed—so far as they were in a position to function when cut off from all nerve connections.

Such a transplant is not in the least like a heart or kidney transplant. A transplanted brain, which carries out no function in the body but just quietly and inscrutably 'thinks its own thoughts', does not signify any progress from a medical point of view. The brain transplant which leads to a close connection between body and brain, which would be considered a far greater sensation than heart transplants, is not likely to come about very soon.

The 'immunity barrier' which has wrecked so many transplants of other organs—the organism's tendency to attack alien bodily tissue as a cause of sickness—is possibly less marked with the brain, it is true, than with heart and kidneys. After the conclusion of his experiments with the transplanted dogs' brains, White found no indication of any damage through an immunological defence reaction of the receiver animal.

That need not mean, however, that a foreign brain would also be tolerated over a longer period, although the brain itself is known to suffer foreign substances readily. Experimenters have deposited skin, fatty tissue, nerve fibres and cancerous growths in the brains of live animals, and such foreign matter has always survived there longer than in any other organ.

The main problem, therefore, facing specialists in organ transplants would perhaps play a smaller rôle with the brain. But other problems, both medical and moral, seem in the long view insoluble. There would, of course, be no difficulty in isolating a live human brain, as White has done with monkeys and dogs. It would even be easier, he says. He has not yet tried it, though he admits he 'would like to study an isolated human brain'. But for the moment he sees no chance of getting such an object of study in his laboratory. 'What family', he sadly asked the journalist Oriana Fallaci, 'would ever authorise me to use a relative from the moment in which his heart stopped? We are locked in traditions, often in the most despicable hypocrisy; one prefers to know that his relative's brain is decaying in the ground rather than to know it's living in a laboratory.'

Various interesting experiments could certainly be carried out with a human brain on a laboratory table, but it is not clear what insights they might bring for a brain transplant. Even the most skilful surgeon is not capable in the available time of attaching all the nerves and blood vessels, which must be cut through in isolating the brain, to the nerves and blood vessel stumps of the proposed receiver, after the latter's dead brain has been cleared out. Even if the impossible were to succeed, the *tour de force* would be useless: the nerve endings once severed would not grow together again.

Assuming the brain could be accommodated in the skull and attached to the receiver's circulation, it would be well provided with blood supply and capable of functioning. But without intact nerve endings it would remain an isolated brain, cut off from its environment, and could not itself make any communication. The brain-receiver's eyes, ears and mouth could not see, hear or say anything, the body would be completely paralysed. The situation would be different, of course, if a surgeon wanted to transplant not only a brain but a whole head. 'That', said White, 'is altogether possible and infinitely easier than isolating a brain as I am doing.' Only relatively few large blood vessels would have to be patched up; but what about the nerves?—the stumps of millions of nerve fibres in the spine could not be united to make them function properly. The person with the new head would remain sectionally paralysed.

Perhaps one day a trick will be discovered to overcome this obstacle as well. But what would be gained by it, and who would benefit? In the last resort, when you think about it, it is quite wrong to talk about a head transplant, for the body without the head is nothing. Our consciousness and our personality are enclosed in the head. Should it ever come to the point that someone's head is combined with someone else's body, then the body will have been transplanted, not the head.

There is a short-story 'black comedy' by Roald Dahl about the brain isolation of an Oxford don with cancer, whose wife blew cigarette smoke in the eye attached to his brain; and in the *Deutsches Ärzteblatt* (German Medical Journal) in 1969 Dr. Bernd Leineweber described the consequences of such a transplant experiment in a science-fiction story. The narrator finds the notebook of a man of fifty-five called Peter Nieburg, who in the first entries complains of troubles with his vision and balance, maddening headaches and symptoms of severe paralysis. He is to have an operation, and reports on this a few days afterwards: 'A young man's head is to be transplanted! I tremble at the idea. What possibilities! Shall I really do it? What shall I think? Shall I think as I would like to, or as my predecessor thought?'

The operation takes place. Soon there are entries from a

student of twenty-five who introduces himself as Klaus Koller, complains at having to make entries in a diary which belongs to one Peter Nieburg, hasn't any idea how he came into the hospital, can only remember jumping from a thirty-foot tower, and is amazed at how old his body has become: 'Grey, flabby!' Bit by bit he learns the truth. With Nieburg's body he is now to continue his life as Nieburg, who lived on his own without relatives. Koller moves into Nieburg's flat and gives himself out to be Nieburg's unknown son. But he cannot come to terms with his body. Continual heart pains intensify his despair: 'I am an old man!' The last entry: 'Have made up my mind. Refuse to bear this filthy fifty-five-year-old body any longer. I shall throw myself in front of a car.'

White's thoughts about this are no different. 'I am a little horrified at the idea of a society in which some men walk about with other men's heads and vice versa.' For the moment there will not be such people, if only because at present the technical difficulties cannot be solved. But something else would already be technically possible today. 'Could a severed human body be kept alive?' Oriana Fallaci asked White, who replied: 'Yes, it isn't difficult. It can be accomplished now with existing techniques.' But he would not be the first to do it. 'I haven't resolved as yet this dilemma: is it right or not?' The Japanese, he thought, would be the first to keep a severed human head in a laboratory.

2

Brain Research Till Modern Times

Long after the human brain had begun to feel curiosity and the exploring urge, it still found the task of self-discovery extremely difficult. Many famous thinkers attributed the work of their brains to other bodily organs, especially the heart and the abdomen; others saw mind and spirit as distributed all over the body. For thousands of years, in fact, man's brightest brains argued about the actual seat of mental activity in the body. Even now it is quite hard to conceive what connection there can be between the wonderland of our impressions and memories, ideas and reflections, emotions, dreams and hopes, and the lumps of soft substance in our brains. We have at our disposal, however, the results of scientific investigations, which no longer leave any doubt as to the brain's importance; they can act as a signpost on the road to discovery. Yet the layman 'still has a mystical conception of the substance of his personal character', wrote Paul Glees, the Göttingen brain researcher, in a recent textbook on the human brain; so he felt he must expressly emphasise his own premises, that 'our mental life is uniquely the organic functioning of the brain'.

The brain was first mentioned in an Egyptian papyrus

which medical historians describe as the oldest surgical manual in the world. This 'Edwin Smith Papyrus' is named after a landowner in upper Egypt concerned with the excavations of 'hundred-gated Thebes', as Homer called the city which for a long time was the centre of the Egyptian empire. Smith bought the papyrus roll, later named after him, in Luxor in 1862. It was about fifty feet long. Investigations showed that it had been written around 1700 B.C., but the medical knowledge it contains certainly comes from a far earlier time, perhaps about a thousand years before that. For Egyptian words appear which were obsolete in 1700 B.C., but were used in the Old Empire.

The main task of the ancient Egyptian surgeons was to treat the injuries arising from accidents and battles. The papyrus contains instructions for this, giving forty-eight cases, their examination and treatment. It is obviously only a fragment, for it begins with the head and ends with the thorax. Twenty-seven of the forty-eight cases are concerned with head injuries, offering detailed descriptions of the wounds suffered by the victims of the hard labour on the pyramids and the battles fought for the glory of the Pharaohs. Here we find the first mention of the brain in extant writings.

In the instructions for treatment of a multiple fracture of the skull (Case 6), it reads:

'If you are examining a man with a gaping head wound which reaches to the bones [and in which] the skull shatters [and] the brain is exposed in the skull, [then] you should feel this wound. [In so doing you find] that the shattered mass of the skull looks like the roughness of melted copper, that something in it throbs [and] flutters under your finger like the soft place on top of a child's skull before it is closed.'

The author of the Smith Papyrus knew that violent action on the skull could have harmful results even when no external injuries could be discovered. He noted that it might lead to the lameness of a leg or to blindness. The papyrus does not show, however, whether the ancient Egyptian doctors had any idea of the brain's unique importance. Probably they did not specially think about it; they accepted the heart as the organ of life and thought. It was the heart which caused argument among the priests and embalmers: should it be left in the body of the departed or taken out? The specialists who prepared corpses for mummification did not bother much with the brain. The widely travelled Greek historian Herodotus (490–c.420 B.C.), who made a thorough study of the Egyptians' methods of embalming, reported: 'They remove with an iron hook as much of the brain as possible through the nostrils. Any of it which the hook cannot get hold of, is washed out by drugs.'

Greece and Alexandria

Greek thinkers who contemplated the seat of the soul reached varying conclusions. Amazingly enough, the earliest investigators came nearest to the facts. Alcmaeon of Croton, for instance, who lived in southern Italy about 500 B.C., decided that the centre for sense perception and thought was in the brain. He dissected animals and was the first to examine the structure of eyes and ears; he discovered that there were nerve paths leading from the sense organs to the brain. He thought of the brain as a gland, which secreted thoughts as the lachrymal gland secreted tears.

'Dr. Hippocrates' (460–377 B.C.), too, considered the founding father of modern medicine, author of the famous Oath, was convinced of the brain's power. 'People should realise', he taught, 'that our pleasures and joys, our laughter and jokes, as also our cares and griefs, our anxiety and tears, come from the brain and only from the brain . . . which is why I assert that the brain is the interpreter of consciousness.' He did not, however, make any investigations into the brain.

So it was open to other philosophers to take a different

view. Democritus (460–371 B.C.), who already conceived of the world as consisting in atoms—the smallest indivisible part-icles—thought that the soul as well as the body was made up of atoms; that these soul atoms were the most mobile of all, and that their motion, which penetrated the whole body, brought about the phenomena of life; they were breathed in with the air, and after death dispersed again into space.

Plato (427–347 B.C.) divided the human soul into three parts: the seat of reason was in the head, and this 'rational soul' was immortal; the irrational soul, subdivided again, was in the body, the higher parts—courage, ambition, and energy—in the heart, the lower—desires, appetite, hunger —in the abdomen. Plato's pupil Aristotle (384–322 B.C.), tutor of the young Alexander the Great, could not go along with his teacher. He saw the heart as the only seat of the soul. All perceptions were taken to the heart as the central organ of the senses; he thought of the brain as a cooling machine for the blood.

The idea of the heart as the centre of the living body, in view of its activity which everybody can feel, seems so obvious that it persisted obstinately over the centuries; and we still meet the relics of this doctrine in use today, when we call someone big-hearted, warm-hearted, hard-hearted, talk about taking something to heart or having a sinking heart. Nor does the cult of the heart survive only in our language; the excitement over the first heart transplants a few years ago was not concerned with the sack of muscle which pumps blood so much as with a mystically transfigured centre of life.

At the time of Aristotle's death no philosopher had made a thorough examination of a human brain. This was first done by Herophilos (c.335–285 B.C.) and Erisistratos (c.310–250 B.C.), two Greek doctors who had come to Alexandria, then the leading trade and cultural centre of the Hellenistic East. Herophilos, called to Alexandria about 300 B.C. to be King Ptolemy I's personal physician, was the first to carry on extensive anatomical studies as well as his medical practice. These investigations, unthinkable till then, were encouraged by his mighty patient, who even allowed him to perform dissections on living people—criminals condemned to death.

He and his younger colleague Erisistratos were specially interested in the brain, and made a great many discoveries. Herophilos described the cerebrum and cerebellum, the meninges, the brain ventricles (cavities). He recognised that the nerves were connected with the brain and the spinal cord; and he transferred the seat of the soul to the brain— the brain ventricles. Erisistratos, studying the brain nerves, made a distinction between sensory and motor nerves. He compared the convolutions of the cerebrum in the human brain to the convolutions in animal brains and, finding the latter less pronounced, concluded: 'The brain in a human being has far more convolutions than in any other living thing, because Man surpasses all in intelligence.'

Dr. Galen and his legacy

The first blossoming of anatomy was quickly over; and for the most part dissections had been only on animals, not men. This was still the case four hundred years later, when animal brains were studied by Galen (129–199 A.D.), a doctor from Asia Minor. His teaching remained the basis for medical thought and action in Europe for fifteen hundred years, and this applied also to his ideas on the importance of the brain.

Born in Pergamum, Galen first served in his home town as a doctor for gladiators, patching up their mangled and shattered bodies. But he soon gave this up, went to Rome, and there quickly achieved the position of the top fashionable doctor, progressing to the post of personal physician to the

Emperor Marcus Aurelius. On the side he was experimenting: he systematically removed different parts of animals'
brains, cut through spinal cord and nerves, and observed
the forms of paralysis which ensued.

Above all, however, he was an indefatigable writer. He
synthesised the various schools and movements in medicine
which had been developed till then, to form a scientific
system which he believed meant the last word in the development of the art of healing. Modesty was not one of his virtues,
and indeed according to the medical historians there are
many other unattractive points in his character. Although
his name meant 'cheerful', 'serene', he was quarrelsome,
vain, ruthless and mendacious, deceiving his pateints and
also claiming the glory for discoveries which were not of his
making.

'So I have carried on my practice into old age,' Galen
declared complacently, 'and till today have nowhere come
to grief in therapy or prognosis, as many other doctors of the
highest repute have done. But if anyone wishes to become
famous in the same way through deeds, not clever talk, he
has only to absorb without trouble what has been established
by me in zealous research throughout my life.'

For about fifty generations this is what doctors did: they
referred to Galen. What he said must be right. His work was
a sort of medical bible.

What did Galen say about the brain and its function?
What were the ideas which kept their attraction for the most
brilliant intellects over many centuries?

Like Plato, he believed in a soul divided into three parts,
with its centres, however, in the liver, the heart and the
brain, all three connected by powers called 'spirit'. The
spiritus naturalis (spirit of nature) in the liver was refined in
the heart to the *spiritus vitalis* (spirit of life). Through the
bloodstream the spirit of life entered the brain, especially
the brain ventricles, where it became the *spiritus animalis* or

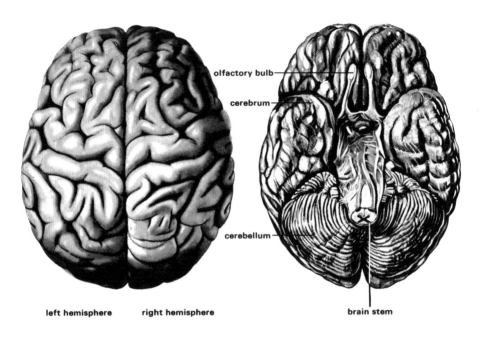

olfactory bulb

cerebrum

cerebellum

brain stem

left hemisphere   right hemisphere

*Anyone looking at a human brain from above (left) sees only the
cerebrum divided into two halves (called hemispheres). But looked at
from below (right), it is obvious that the brain has no uniform
structure.*

pneuma psychicon (soul-spirit), an air-like noble substance
so thin and mobile that it could itself flow through the finest
nerves. Galen thought of the nervous system as a system of
pipes. By contracting and expanding again, the brain
pumped the soul-spirit from the brain ventricles, a reservoir
for this thin substance, into the nerve pipes.

We can no longer feel the fascination of this doctrine. The
reason why it was accepted till the seventeenth century has
been described by Karl Rothschuh, director of the Institute
for the History of Medicine at the University of Münster:

'It is partly because the spirit theory provided an explanation for a whole series of phenomena, like the perception disorders and motor paralyses when nerves are severed, psychological disorders after brain damage, and also fainting, sleep and related phenomena. Secondly, Galen's teaching on the nerves was only part of a great unified system of medicine, which looked extremely fixed (because its anatomical and physiological foundations and the teaching about illness based on them seemed so solid); with the result that no one could easily wean himself from such a system. Thirdly, Galen's spirit doctrine fitted in beautifully with the Christian idea of the soul. We should remember that the Middle Ages did not feel the urge, as later ages did, to carry out new investigations; there was quite enough to do absorbing and interpreting what had been handed down by the ancient doctor.'

The last remains of the spirit doctrine could still be found in the scientific works of the nineteenth century. But only outsiders took this attitude; most brain researchers had long been converted to other ideas, even though many of these were no nearer the truth.

The progress of anatomy

The turning-point in brain research came in 1543, when Andreas Vesalius, the founder of modern anatomy, a teacher in Padua, published the first anatomy book based on precise new observations and not on Galen's writings. He pointed out many mistakes in Galen's work, and also doubted whether the brain ventricles played as important a part as Galen had thought. In his view—already much nearer the facts— the soul-spirit came up in the grey cortex of the cerebrum and the cerebellum.

Since then many anatomists have been extensively concerned with the brain. They have dissected thousands of human brains, belonging to young and old, men and women, sick and healthy, members of all races. They have weighed and measured brains and also—not very profitably—tried to find connections between each brain's weight, measurements and appearance and the mental achievements of its late owner.

The human brain, as the early anatomists already saw, consists of various parts. Admittedly, looked at from above or from the side, it appears homogeneous, like a walnut kernel with its twisted fissures. Seen from below, however, it shows a collection of knotty excrescences, which quickly put out of mind the walnut image. With this perspective it appears like a conglomeration of various organs which, although they work closely together, have separate functions to attend to. This appearance, indeed, as it gradually transpired, is also reality.

Like a rope about the thickness of a finger, the spinal cord leads from below into the brain. It merges imperceptibly into the medulla oblongata, the lowest region of a sphere of the brain with three parts which anatomists call the brain stem. The other parts are the corpus callosum, a swelling clearly set off from the medulla oblongata, and the mid-brain.

From the brain stem the cerebellum sticks out behind. Its surface is densely and deeply furrowed. It consists of two halves projecting to left and right, but not completely separate from each other.

Above the brain stem lies the diencephalon with the two areas called thalamus and hypothalamus. Below the hypothalamus, hanging by a thin stalk, is the pituitary gland (hypophysis), little bigger than a pea, which because of its close connection with the brain is the most influential hormonal gland in the body.

The cerebrum with its furrowed surface vaults over all sections of the brain. It is in fact large compared to them, making up four-fifths of the human brain. A deep cleft separates the right and left halves of the cerebrum from each

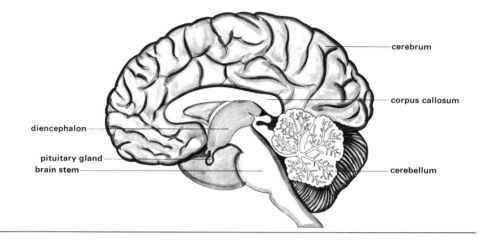

Longitudinal section of a human brain.

1817264

other. The bottom of the cleft forms the corpus callosum, a massive cord of nerve fibres, which connects together the two halves of the cerebrum.

The brain mass with its different sections, which is rather soft and therefore sensitive to shock, is housed in the skull with amazing safety. Three meninges (membranes) protect the brain from shocks which meet the skull. The 'dura mater' of tough fibres lines the brain ventricles and so pads the hard bones. Further in is the fine arachnoid (spider's web); and for a third covering the soft 'pia mater' nestles close to the surface of the cerebrum. Between the arachnoid and the pia flows the cerebrospinal fluid; this lymph-like brain fluid also circulates through the ventricles of the brain in a single interconnected system.

Anatomists distinguished a great many more structures in the brain. Brains were cut up into the thinnest of slices.

Millimetre by millimetre researchers investigated specimens of the brain first under the light microscope, later under the electron microscope as well. Observations on patients with sick or damaged brains promoted new knowledge about man's master organ, as did systematic investigations on animals of many kinds. Surgical operations brought surprising discoveries. Researchers extracted secrets from the brain by stimulating it with slight electric shocks. They exposed it to the deliberate influence of chemical substances, made it sleep in the service of science and intervened in its dreams.

Galen's long-lived spirit theory was followed by a doctrine of 'nerve sap'. Then it was a 'nerve force' which the brain was supposed to keep going; till finally it was established that electric currents circulated in the brain. It is electric signals which enable the brain to come into connection with other parts of the body. But closely connected with the brain's electrical activity there are complex chemical processes which today many brain researchers are occupied in elucidating.

For a long time now brain research has split up into many special fields. Sometimes there is so much interest in detail that a view of the functioning of the whole is blurred. Many ideas about how the brain works are still provisional, and even today errors are quite possible. But at least, unlike Galen's spirit doctrine, they no longer have the chance of congealing into a dogma.

For, like any modern science, present-day brain research is distinguished by the fact that old theories have continually to be tested against new findings. If they do not pass these tests, they are rejected.

3

The Split Brain

Man has two arms and legs, two lungs and kidneys, eyes and ears—but only one heart and brain. Still, the heart consists of equal halves, even though their form is not exactly symmetrical; and the brain is also divided into two halves, which are almost symmetrical.

Many massive fibre bundles join the two sides of the brain. In man, the largest of these commissures (linking pathways) is the corpus callosum which connects the 'hemispheres', the two halves of the cerebral cortex. What would happen if the corpus callosum were severed, isolating the right and left hemispheres?

This is just what has been done by American scientists with cats and monkeys, and doctors have carried out the operation on men. The findings which have come from such operations are among the most exciting in modern brain research. At first sight, when the patients had recovered from the operation, they appeared unaltered, showing no changes in their temperament, personality or intelligence. But special tests revealed a sensational fact: people with split brains react as if they had two brains functioning independently and without any knowledge of each other.

The function of the corpus callosum in the brain had long been a puzzle for scientists. Brain surgeons who sometimes could not help cutting into it during operations were amazed at the lack of apparent harmful effects on their patients. At the end of the 'thirties they discovered, also with surprise, that the severing of the corpus callosum even had a beneficial effect on epileptics subject to very frequent severe fits. But this did not do anything to explain the importance of the corpus callosum for the functioning of the brain. In 1951 the neurophysiologist Warren S. McCulloch of Yale University wrily asserted that its only function seemed to consist in promoting the transference of epileptic fits from one half of the body to the other. There was the same flavour of bafflement in the jocular comment by another American authority, Professor Karl S. Lashley, that the purpose of the corpus callosum must be 'to keep the two hemispheres from caving in'.

A first indication of its real function was discovered in the early 'fifties by Ronald Myers in the course of his doctoral thesis which he started at the University of Chicago and continued at the California Institute of Technology. He was experimenting with a cat whose corpus callosum he had severed. He observed that the cat was no longer capable of transferring what it had just learnt from one hemisphere to the other.

In his experiments he first bandaged its left eye and made it learn with the right eye to distinguish two signs, a square and a circle. It was only rewarded if it pressed a panel on which a square was drawn. Directly the cat had mastered its lesson, he bandaged the other eye, and took off the previous bandage. The cat was now to show what it had just learnt by way of the right eye. But with its split brain it could no longer carry out a task which is no problem at all for cats with undamaged brains. The lesson was not stored in both hemispheres, as is usually the case, but only in the right one.

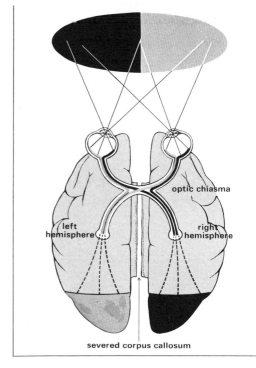

The visual impressions from the left half of the visual field come into the right hemisphere, visual impressions from the right half of the visual field into the left hemisphere. Since the corpus callosum is severed, the two hemispheres cannot exchange the information received.

This may need some amplification. Each hemisphere normally has specific control over one side of the body— the opposite side: the left hemisphere controls the right side, and vice versa. With the eyes, things are rather more complicated. From each eye an optic nerve with many nerve fibres conducts all visual impressions to the brain. Where the two optic nerves meet, they join to exchange half of their fibres: the fibres from the right half of each retina go to the right hemisphere, those of the left half of the retina to the left hemisphere. This seems to be in contradiction to the principle that each hemisphere controls the other side of the body; but in fact the left half of the retina in each eye attends to all impressions in the right half of the visual field, and the other way round with the right half of the retina. So in the end the visual impressions absorbed by both eyes from the left half of the visual field enter the right hemisphere, the other way round with the impressions absorbed in the right half of the visual field.

With Myers's cat, besides the corpus callosum, the intersection of the optic nerves (optic chiasma) had also been severed so that each hemisphere was only connected with one eye, the eye on the same side. So the right hemisphere learned what the right eye had seen, and as there was no connection with the left hemisphere, it had to keep its knowledge to itself; and the left hemisphere had to learn its task on its own.

In another experiment Myers made each hemisphere of a cat's brain learn different things. The right one learned that the key with the square meant a reward and the key with the circle drew a blank; the left one had exactly the opposite implanted. The cat with split brain found no difficulty in learning such contradictory matter, whereas cats with intact corpus callosum become neurotic if faced with such a situation.

Discoveries on W.J.

Myers, his supervisor Roger W. Sperry, and a host of colleagues, made extensive investigations of the results of brain-splitting in cats and monkeys, until the opportunity arose in 1961 to carry out such studies on a man. (Studies on men had been carried out in the 'forties but with little success.) The man in question was a war invalid aged forty-eight, in Los Angeles, with brain damage; the doctors revealed only his initials, W.J. He was the first man with severed hemispheres on whom the consequences of the operation were thoroughly studied.

As a result of his war injury W.J. had been subject to severe epileptic fits up to ten times a day. None of the drugs by which epileptics can often be freed from fits had brought relief. So he accepted a proposal by neurosurgeons that he should have the corpus callosum severed. After the operation his fits disappeared almost completely. Otherwise nothing seemed to have changed with W.J., described as being above average in intelligence. 'In a casual conversation over a cup of coffee and a cigarette,' Sperry reported, 'one would hardly suspect there was anything at all unusual about him.'

On systematic investigation, however, a simple test was enough to reveal a divergence from the norm. Michael S. Gazzaniga, now of New York University, who was then one of Sperry's team, made W.J. close his eyes, put into his right hand an easily identifiable object, like a pencil, spoon or banana, and asked him: What have you got in your hand? W.J. answered without hesitation as anyone else would do. But when Gazzaniga put the same object into his left hand, he could not say what it was.

Gazzaniga, the first scientist to observe this phenomenon, found it easy enough to explain. Both hemispheres, besides their competence for the opposite side of the body, have special functions to fulfil as well. With all right-handed and most left-handed people—and with W.J.—the left hemisphere contains the speech centre. Though the right hemisphere could register what the left hand was holding, it could not make its owner speak about this. To do so, it would have needed co-operation with the speech-skilled left hemisphere, with which there was now no connection.

That the mute hemisphere knew exactly what the left hand had felt was shown by another test. When W.J. was invited to show on a blackboard the object he had just held in his left hand, he carried this out without difficulty. But he could point to the picture only with his left hand. For only the right hemisphere, which controls the left hand, could know what the left hand had felt.

Tests for the hemispheres

The good result of the brain-splitting operation in fighting epileptic fits encouraged neurosurgeons to make the incision into the corpus callosum for other patients liable to such fits which were otherwise not susceptible to influence. The patients, impressed by the improvements reached, agreed very readily to be further subjects for Gazzaniga's research; so he was able to undertake a series of extremely interesting experiments.

With the help of split-brain patients he discovered that the right hemisphere, although not having like the left a speech centre, was not unintelligent or even completely incapable of speech. In one experiment he made his subjects look at a point exactly in the centre of a screen. Then he projected the word 'pencil' on to the left half of the visual field. So long as the subjects gazed fixedly straight ahead, only the right hemisphere could register this information. Then he put a pencil with some other objects in front of the patients, and asked them, without looking, to pick out with their left hand the object named; they duly reached for the pencil. The right hemisphere, he observed, could even put together words from large plastic letters. A subject with his eyes closed placed simple words like 'love' or 'cup'—but could not say what he had just spelt: the left hemisphere, needed for speech, did not know what the left hand had spelt.

Gazzaniga projected on to the screen before his subjects the word 'heart', so that the first two letters were to be read in the left part of the visual field, the last three in the right part. Asked what was on the screen, the subjects immediately said 'art'. But when invited to pick out with the left hand from among several cards the card on which the word stood, they pointed to 'he'.

Although mute, therefore, the right hemisphere had its own vocabulary, but this was limited. Gazzaniga discovered no support for the theory that it understood verbs. If he projected the word 'smile' or 'frown' on the left side of the screen—which only the right hemisphere could perceive if the subjects gazed straight ahead—they showed no reaction. This hemisphere also proved weak in grammar: the subjects could not form the plural of words which they had put

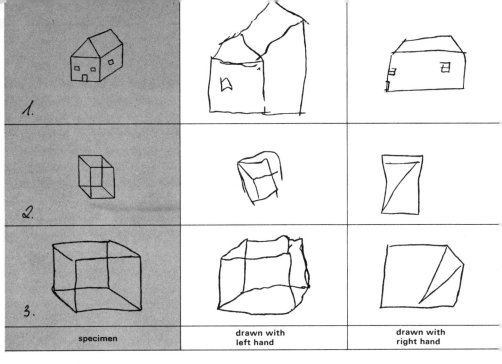

	drawn with left hand	drawn with right hand
specimen		

Tests on patients with split brains showed that the right hemisphere is superior to the left in perspective drawing. Although the patient who did the drawings in the middle and right column is right-handed, he could only carry out the tasks set him with the left hand (which is controlled by the right hemisphere).

together from plastic letters with their left hand.

But the right hemisphere had capacities lacked by the left despite its speech powers. The sense of forms and spatial structures was much more pronounced in the right hemisphere than in the left. Drawings of a house or a cube, perfect in perspective, were possible only with the left hand, not the right, even though the subjects were right-handed.

Gazzaniga was amazed at how skilfully the subjects covered up the effects produced by severance of the hemispheres. This skill was also the explanation of the fact that doctors had previously not observed any striking differences in patients with split brains.

For instance, he projected on to the left of the screen a

succession of green and red lights. The subject had to say each time which light had just come up. The task was actually insoluble; for only the right hemisphere (without the power of speech) registered the lights. But after a short time the subject regularly gave the correct colour—leaving Gazzaniga rather disturbed. Eventually he hit on the trick. The left hemisphere first made a guess. Assuming the right hemisphere saw red light and the left guessed 'green', the right heard the answer spoken out loud, and since it had registered red light, it could not agree and caused a head-shake. The left took this as a sign that it had guessed wrong, and corrected itself, making the subject quickly say 'red'. If the left had guessed correctly first time, then there was no head-shake.

Both hemispheres were capable of emotional reactions. This was established by Gazzaniga during the experiments when he unexpectedly projected on to the screen among other pictures the photograph of a naked girl. The split-brain subjects gave amused grins, regardless of whether the nude was presented to the left or the right hemisphere. But if it appeared in the left half of their visual field and so could only be registered by the right hemisphere, they couldn't say what they really found so funny. One female subject, when it was presented to her right hemisphere, even stated that she did not see anything at all; and in fact the left hemisphere with the power of speech did not see anything. As against that—she giggled: the reaction of the right hemisphere. Gazzaniga asked what was amusing her. The left hemisphere, having no idea, at first showed embarrassment, then pretended it knew: 'Oh, that funny thing!'

Two working brains

'All the evidence indicates'—Gazzaniga concluded from his experiments—'that separation of the hemispheres creates

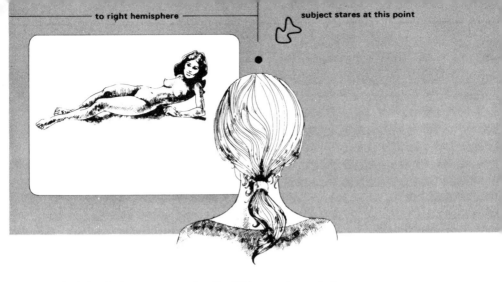

Both hemispheres react emotionally. This was shown during tests on patients with split brains who were unexpectedly shown the picture of a naked girl.

two independent spheres of consciousness within a single cranium, that is to say within a single organism.'

This conclusion was supported by an experiment also carried out at the University of California. A monkey's corpus callosum was severed, with the optic chiasma cut through in such a way that—contrary to the natural conditions—only one eye supplied each hemisphere with visual impressions. A leucotomy, an operation leading to extreme indifference (see Chapter 6), was carried out on one hemisphere. A blinker was used to allow the monkey to see with only one eye at a time. At first the free eye was the one which supplied the intact hemisphere with information. The experimenter showed the monkey a snake, and it promptly reacted as monkeys tend to react if they see a snake: it took fright and wanted to run away. The experimenter then took off the blinker and tied it over the other eye, after which he repeated the experiment, presenting the snake to the hemisphere which had been operated on. This time the monkey remained calm. Under the control of the hemisphere which had been rendered indifferent, the snake made no impression on it at all. It seemed as if the body were governed by two different personalities.

Not all the authorities, however, agree with Gazzaniga that 'cross-cueing' is always the explanation of how one hemisphere gains 'impossible' knowledge from the other; or with his conclusion that two independent spheres of consciousness can reside in one body. Some people find this disturbing, he says, because they look on consciousness as an indivisible quality of the human brain. Others find the conclusion premature because they feel that the capacities of the right hemisphere revealed so far lie at the level of an automaton. The former objection is perhaps a relic of a traditional mystical conception, which is becoming less and less tenable with the results of modern brain research; the latter is unconvincing in view of the fact that phenomena of recognition, action and learning take place independently in both hemispheres under certain experimental conditions, and that even though they are relatively primitive activities they can clearly be the basis for thought processes, that is well beyond the automaton level.

At any rate the results of experiments with split-brain animals and men are acknowledged everywhere. Soon there should be further results available, and this will lead to greater unity in interpreting the whole complex of split-brain problems.

Advantages of splitting brains?

For those who are mainly interested in the practical effects of research findings, of course, this is only the beginning of the story of the split brains. Till now it was a new method of research which made it possible to help a very small circle of sick people and thereby to achieve important discoveries about our brain. A very much wider application of the brain-splitting operation is now conceivable, as

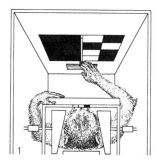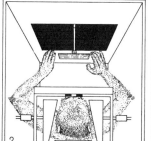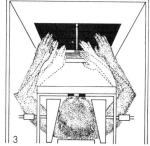

Higher performance with split brains? Monkeys, whose hemispheres had been severed by researchers, carried out specific tasks better than monkeys with brains intact. In this task the monkeys had to tap on panels which had lit up for the fraction of a second, making as few mistakes as possible.

Gazzaniga has indicated: 'It is altogether possible that if a human brain is divided very early in life, the two hemispheres, separated and independently of each other, might develop intellectual functions of a high order, at a level which can be reached by normal people only in the left hemisphere.'

For the researchers at California Institute of Technology, the first thing was to investigate whether animals and men with split brains were capable of processing more information than those of their species with intact brains.

To investigate this with monkeys, they constructed a special test stand. The monkeys had first to pull a handle, on which eight of sixteen panels briefly lit up for them. The test was for them to press with both hands on as many as possible of the panels which had lit up.

Monkeys with intact brains pressed three-quarters of the right panels when the panels were lit for 600 milliseconds. Split-brain monkeys pressed all the right panels when these were lit for only 200 milliseconds. Their optic chiasma had been severed, and firmly fixed spectacles made them cover exactly eight panels with each eye.

Split-brain men also proved superior at such tasks to people with undivided brains. 'We have found', Gazzaniga reported, 'that patients with split brains can carry out two tasks as quickly as a normal person can master one.' The split-brain patients scarcely made any use of this superiority; for the problems set them were of a kind which do not come up much in daily life!—and they were adapted to the performance capacity of the 'unintelligent' and inarticulate right hemisphere. But assuming that this, too, could have intelligence and differentiated speech potential, might not a split brain be of practical use?

This idea is more than pure fancy. With lower mammals, and even up to monkeys, both hemispheres are equal: not only externally symmetrical, but also in their functions. With men, however, differentiated speech, which distinguishes us from animals, has settled by preference in one hemisphere, the left one for the vast majority of all humans.

Until the results of the latest research, it was generally thought that we are born with our brains still symmetrical, and that during the first year of life the speech functions become tied to the left hemisphere, although at that stage the brain still reacts flexibly. Evidence seemed to show that if the whole of the left hemisphere had to be removed because of an intolerable or potentially fatal illness, the right hemisphere immediately learned to speak; but that if a child had already reached school age when a removal of the left hemisphere became unavoidable, the consequences were far harder to overcome.

The American scientist J. A. Wada has recently observed that even in prematurely born babies, in most cases, certain parts of the left temporal lobe are larger than comparable areas on the right hemisphere; they are parts associated with language. This finding, if confirmed, would suggest that the left hemisphere is genetically 'pre-set' to control language.

Even if the theory about babies were true, the situation is evidently not hopeless even with adults. In 1966 neurosurgeons at the University of Nebraska reported on a patient of forty-seven who, after removal of the left hemisphere, had learnt to speak, sing, write and read again.

The most amazing thing is that the lack of a hemisphere, especially when it has been removed at a very early age, appears to make little difference to the patient, once he has recovered from the serious operation. This raises the question whether we do not use our brains all too little, if we can dispense so easily with one half of them. Here is where Gazzaniga's speculation comes in: could the right hemisphere be made to develop like the left if the two were severed from each other early enough? Supposing that splitting a baby's brain had such an effect, would it really be an advantage to have a brain with both sides good for thought and speech? Would the equalised hemispheres, thinking independently, complement each other to produce undreamt-of mental achievements, or would they—like the executives of many business firms—use up a large part of thinking capacity merely in intriguing for power?

No one is yet thinking of splitting babies' brains. But it is quite conceivable that new discoveries by brain researchers may bring nearer this possibility of manipulation.

There is another consequence to be drawn from the studies of brain-splitting: they show that ideas for educating children may be urgently in need of revision. Observations on split-brain patients have shown that the right hemisphere is superior to the left where what is needed is not knowledge communicated by articulateness and speech, but rather practical intelligence. The education of children today, however, is almost entirely orientated towards transmitting knowledge grasped in words: they are supposed to learn through textbooks and through teachers talking. There is very little provision for transmitting knowledge through their own practical activity or even their own ideas.

Might this be why the right hemisphere works so poorly compared with the left? Has it remained backward simply because it does not get enough attention with our kind of education? Perhaps the only reason why it does not come up just as impressively with practical abilities as the left hemisphere with its skill in speech and expressiveness is that we let it atrophy. Roger Sperry, who with his colleagues started on the brain-splitting studies, is convinced that the right hemisphere is neglected in many countries' educational systems, and that this is a great disadvantage. He pleads for training in practical abilities to be given far more attention in schools than it is today.

4

The Evolution of the Brain

'And the earth was waste and void,' it says in Genesis. Twenty-five verses and six days later the work was finished: 'And God created man in his image.' Even the strictest fundamentalist would no doubt accept that it took rather longer than six days to reach the crown of creation. The discoveries of science show that over three thousand million years have passed in gradual evolution from the simplest form of life before man arose with his unique speciality in the realm of living things: his brain.

There were brains long before that, of course. About four hundred million years ago, even before the first vertebrates evolved, there were creatures with brains: rudimentary nervous systems go back still further into the primitive history of life. Through comparative studies of the brains of species still extant today at various stages of evolution, biologists have been able to trace the evolution of the brain from the simplest connecting systems between nerve cells to the thinking and animated marvel in our head which has conscious experience of its environment.

Unicellular animals have no nervous system, but they too are already concerned with communication: they register what is happening on their outer surface. The membrane surrounding the cell content is responsive to stimuli, which are transmitted to all parts of the cell body.

When the protozoa, first forms of life, joined up to become multicellular organisms, this soon led to cells being developed with the special function of receiving and transmitting stimuli: nerve cells. Only the sponges, lowest form of multicellular organisms, are without any nerve cells. The next form higher than that, the coelenterates, which include, for instance, jelly-fish and polyps, already have a simple nervous system. Their bodies are covered with a net of nerve cells with long fibres. A stimulus meeting any part of the body is transmitted to all parts of the organism, on which the body reacts only as a whole: it contracts and carries out oscillations or wave-like movements.

With flat-worms the arrangement of the nervous system is more elaborate. This development, it is clear, was closely connected with a new feature in the structural plan which was kept from then on in the animal kingdom right up to man: the flat-worm's body, like man's, is symmetrically built, with a right and left side exactly reflecting each other for the whole length of the body. So with this innovation went an improvement in the nervous system. Flat-worms' nerve cells are concentrated in two cords which go through the body from front to back. At intervals they branch off into nerves which receive stimuli from the section of the body near to each nerve, and also transmit stimuli to it.

Isaac Asimov of Boston University illustrated the advances achieved by the flat-worm with an impressive analogy. The nervous system of the coelenterates, he said, was like a telephone exchange where all subscribers are attached to a single connection, so that if anyone calls another subscriber, the 'phone rings for all subscribers; whereas with flat-worms it was like an exchange where a caller directly reaches the person he is calling, and only that person.

A bilaterally symmetrical creature, usually longer than it

is wide, is inclined to move 'longitudinally', which results in the formation of specialised front and rear ends. Clearly, sense organs are best placed in the front part of an extended body, and as the front end reaches food first, a mouth opening in front is also extremely useful. Such a development was bound to have effects on the nervous system. With the evolution of a part of the head, nerve cells became concentrated in the front end of the body. Even in flat-worms the nerve cords at the head end are bigger and better formed than those in the rest of the body. Biologists see the primacy of the head part within the nervous system as the beginnings of brain development.

So the animal kingdom has a brain, from the worms onward. Nor apparently are the concentrations of nerve cells in the heads of invertebrates completely exhausted by the processing of sense stimuli and the tasks of control and co-ordination. For zoologists have succeeded in training even worms to do very simple tricks. Octopi (a stage higher in evolution) proved capable of distinguishing various geometrical patterns.

Space for intelligence

A remarkable development of the brain started with the vertebrates—called, of course, after the vertebrae which surround the main nerve cord, the spinal cord. Till then all creatures, like the flat-worms, had a double nerve cord going through the body on the belly side. This was unprotected unless the creature had an outer skeleton, as was the case, for instance, with mussels, crabs or beetles. Another new thing with vertebrates was the bony case round the brain, the skull.

Even in the brains of the most primitive vertebrates, biologists distinguish three parts which appear as bladder-shaped swellings: 'hind brain', 'mid-brain' and 'fore-brain'.

These differentiated further in the course of evolution to additional parts of the brain, the hind brain turning into the brain stem and cerebellum, the fore-brain into the diencephalon and cerebrum.

The brains of the two lowest classes of vertebrates, fishes and amphibians, were still not very impressive. But with reptiles two tendencies showed up clearly: brains became bigger, and the cerebrum grew in proportion to the whole. Biologists connect this development with the transition to living on land, which makes more demands on the brain than an aquatic life.

The more powerful brains provided a condition for the emergence of larger species of reptile; but obviously owing to insufficient co-ordination, this led to excessive physical size. The gigantic dinosaurs of the Mesozoic Era had tiny brains. The stegosaurus, thirty feet long, a massive mountain of flesh, its spine covered with great sharp ridges of bone like a comb, possessed a brain no bigger than a cat's today. It was not enough to control the mighty body, so the creature had a second brain at the bottom end of the spinal cord, which was bigger, in fact, than the brain at the head end.

This principle evidently did not persist. The saurians died out, and the smaller reptile species evolved into the first mammals. Creatures the size of shrews became the primitive ancestors of the most successful class of vertebrates which eventually ruled the earth. The mammals could achieve a dominating position because, this time, the brain kept in step with the increasing physical size. Mammal brains became so spacious that the routine tasks which occurred in the body's organisational headquarters left room for functions which in the widest sense could be called intelligence.

This development reached its climax in the mammalian order of primates, to which man also belongs. The primates first branched off as an inconspicuous group of 'insect-eaters', a group which today includes shrews, hedgehogs and moles.

Most primates, like monkeys and lemurs, are tree-dwellers and have prehensile hands and feet. Their stay in the trees, which demands of the brain a more precise co-ordination of bodily movements than does life on the ground, and the development of prehensile limbs, gave the crucial incentives, in the opinion of many scientists, for the evolution of more powerful brains. The primates evolved into brain-animals, with man far surpassing all the others in this class.

The weight of the brain in anthropoid apes, man's nearest relatives, is only about a third of the average human brain. Among these apes the gorilla has the largest brain; but as it has to serve a massive body, the much smaller chimpanzee with its somewhat lighter brain is more intelligent.

Considering the long intervals otherwise in the evolution of life, it is incredible in how short a time the expansion of the brain distinguishing man from the anthropoid apes has taken place. The gorilla's brain fills a skull space of about thirty cubic inches. With the various finds of extinct hominids, today brought together as a species called *Homo erectus,* calculations produced a skull content of as much as fifty-four cubic inches. The time when *Homo erectus* spread over Africa, Asia and Europe is not very far back: the oldest remains of this extinct hominid are a million years old, the most recent half a million. But since then the brain has again grown enormously: present-day man has a brain on average of about eighty-four cubic inches. The impulse for this extraordinary giant growth of brain is in doubt, but the result is known. It made man the lord of creation, capable of carrying out the idea of God in Genesis: 'Replenish the earth and subdue it.' It also allowed him to carry out this demand so thoroughly that his survival is threatened today by his own actions. Man's brain did not stop him drifting to the brink of self-destruction.

Somewhere on the way from the primates, with their less luxuriant brains, to man came the development of the mental abilities and spiritual qualities which man specially

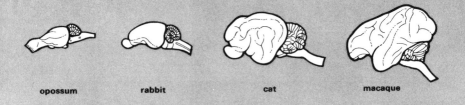

opossum   rabbit   cat   macaque

Between the brain of man and of his closest relative in the animal kingdom, the chimpanzee, the difference in size is more marked than between a chimpanzee brain and a brain of lower mammals (all the brains are drawn to the correct scale).

values in himself; and also perhaps consciousness. Even more puzzling than the sudden enlargement of the brain is the question of what conditions were needed in brain evolution for the emergence of the human mind, Descartes's *Cogito, ergo sum.* Why can man think?

It cannot be simply a matter of the brain's size. Both elephants and whales have far bigger brains. While the weight of a human brain is between three and four pounds, elephant brains may weigh eleven pounds, and whale brains even more. Both are clever animals, but their mental powers are not up to man's! Scientists have argued that they need more brain mass because they have a very much bigger body than man. If one reckons how many tens of pounds of body have to be controlled by how many pounds of brain, man comes out much better—but this calculation raises another problem. Mice show a similar proportion to man between brain weight and body weight; sparrows an even better one. So what about the proverbial 'sparrow brain'?

Smaller animals obviously need relatively more brain than larger ones as 'basic equipment'. On this principle new calculations were made. The Basle zoologist Adolf Portmann

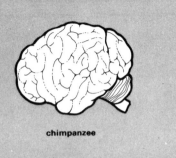
chimpanzee

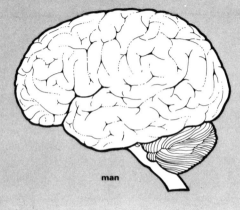
man

started from the premise that each vertebrate's brain had an 'elementary apparatus' in the brain stem, a piece of basic equipment which he called the stem residue. Portmann determined the smallest possible residue for mammals of various sizes and then divided the weight of the 'higher integration sorts' of brain, in the essential cerebrum, cerebellum and diencephalon, by the weight of the stem residue corresponding to the size of each animal.

In this way he obtained for each mammal a standard which he called a 'pallium index' so that in comparing various brains the differences in body sizes were taken into account. For man he worked out a pallium index of 170, against only 2 for mice, 49 for chimpanzees, 104 for the Indian elephant. But dolphins, although he could not make exact calculations, he assessed at nearly 120, their near relatives, pig-whales, at 150 to 160.

By this reckoning the human brain is again not so far superior as one would think to the brains of other mammals. Perhaps the pallium index fails to do justice to the special qualities of the human brain (and also puts the chimpanzee brain at a disadvantage); or are dolphins and whales really endowed with far greater mental powers than most people suppose?

The American neurologist John C. Lilly has long been trying to find out more about dolphins, especially through attempts to decipher their language, which consists of a great variety of sounds. He is convinced that in about a decade man will reach possibilities of communication with the dolphins far beyond what is common in conditioning for circus tricks. It remains to be seen whether this hope is fulfilled, and what will come of our new inter-species understanding—shall we yet see dolphin philosophers?

5

Charting the Cortex

The patient was fully conscious, and knew exactly where she was: in the operating theatre of the Neurological Institute at the University of Montreal. Wilder Penfield, one of the most famous neurosurgeons not only in Canada but in the world, was operating on the left hemisphere of her brain to cure her of severe epileptic fits.

He had opened the skull and was talking to his patient, who had been given only a local anaesthetic for his sole object was to banish the pain caused by penetrating the scalp and the cranium. The brain is insensitive to touch, and even drastic operations produce no feeling of pain.

To investigate the operation area, Penfield stimulated various places in the exposed cerebrum with slight electrical current. Suddenly the woman cried: 'I hear my mother and my brother talking to each other.' When he stopped the stimulation, she told him what she had just heard and also seen: mother and brother had been talking in the sitting-room at home, and she had been there. Everything was as if it had really happened, although she also knew at the time that she was in the theatre at the Neurological Institute and was having an operation.

Penfield has reported on many similar observations. Under the influence of the electric current one patient heard an orchestra play, another re-experienced the birth of her child. A young man saw and heard his cousin in South Africa laugh and speak. A patient had the impression he was standing 'at the corner of Jacob Street and Worthington Street in South Bend, Indiana'. A mother heard her young son calling in the yard outside her kitchen, and also registered the other noises which somehow belonged to the scene, car horns, dogs barking, children shouting. A woman from Holland re-experienced in the operating theatre something which had moved her very deeply years before: she felt she was in church in her home town on Christmas Eve, heard the carols, and was much affected by the solemnity of the illusory scene.

Events which had really taken place in the past were continually being electrically conjured up, although as a rule the patients had not thought about these experiences for a long time. Nor did the experiences, often quite ordinary and insignificant, seem good material for the psycho-analyst. They were different from mere recollection not only in their 'realism' and the feeling they gave of direct participation; they also took place in a characteristic way. 'When the neurosurgeon's electrode accidentally activates a past event,' Penfield writes, 'that event unfolds continuously, moment by moment. It is a little like the playing of a tape or running of a filmstrip, which has on it all the things a person once registered—the things which he has selected by his attention in the period concerned.' This filmstrip from a long-forgotten time always ran forwards, never backwards— nor were there any flash-backs. And it ran all the time the current was flowing at the same place in the brain. 'There is no pausing, no turning back, no overlapping with other events,' Penfield reported. 'If the electrode is withdrawn, it stops just as suddenly as it began.'

When the electric stimulation was resumed at the same

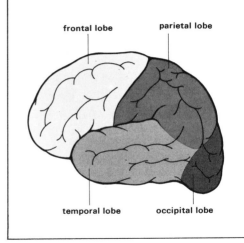

Brain researchers have subdivided each hemisphere into four 'lobes'.

frontal lobe   parietal lobe

temporal lobe   occipital lobe

place after a brief interruption, the same filmstrip sometimes began to run again. The experience, however, did not go on from where it was broken off, but started from the beginning.

Such experiences can be activated only in certain parts of the cerebrum above the ears, the 'temporal lobes'. For better orientation and understanding, brain-researchers have subdivided each hemisphere into four lobes: frontal lobes, parietal lobes, temporal and occipital lobes. Some of the boundaries are formed by marked fissures between the brain convolutions; others seem arbitrarily defined. As has been said, the cerebrum, seen from above, looks a unified whole, but this is a false impression.

The man who in the 1930s made the first observations of 'filmstrip experiences' must be given the credit for many discoveries on the functioning of various parts of the brain. Penfield, in fact, became one of the most successful researchers in charting the human cerebrum and investigating which regions were responsible for which tasks.

Dr. Gall and the phrenologists

The idea that there was a division of labour in the brain first came to Dr. Franz Joseph Gall, who was born in 1758 near Pforzheim and later practised in Vienna and Paris.

Having carried out anatomical studies of the human brain, he recognised that the white substance which made up the largest part of the cerebrum consisted of fibres, and that the origin of these fibres lay in the grey substance only a few millimetres thick, which formed the surface of the cerebrum, the cerebral cortex.

Against the opinion of weighty authorities of his time Gall maintained that the cerebral cortex was of supreme importance for mental life. He saw the cerebrum as the material basis for all intellectual and moral activity; and believed that every phenomenon of mental life had its special seat in the brain. He collected hundreds of human and animal skulls, had wax moulds made of skulls and wax preparations of brains, and completed his museum with wax masks of contemporaries known and unknown. In his enthusiasm over the theory that various human qualities could be localised in the brain, the head-hunter made untenable assertions by which, however, many people were fascinated.

To an increasingly ardent band of disciples he proclaimed that a man's mental and spiritual faculties could be recognised by the shape of the head. If a region of the cortex were particularly well developed, this would lead to prominences in the corresponding part of the skull, and observations on such prominences would reveal individual differences in human faculties. A high forehead, he taught, was a sign of intellectual ability and powers of judgement, a long back of the head showed loyalty and devotion. Matrimonial and sexual instincts, and sexual love, were located in the neck; there were faculties of prudence, modesty and reserve, of self-esteem and ambition, of mimicry and of wit, of high (religious) feelings, aggressiveness, attraction to wine and to food.

'Here in Paris,' he wrote complacently to a friend in 1827:

'collections of human and animal skulls or moulages (moulds) are made in all the academies. And those who in the early days were shouting so loud about the 'charlatan', are obliged to accept the reality of my observations. All over England there are large societies concerned with these investigations who will see that justice is done to the discoverers. The doctrine has spread right to Calcutta. So you see, my friend, that I can consider myself justified in making a claim to distinguished heads, including yours. My collection is expanding daily . . .'

Gall's skull doctrine, called phrenology (after the Greek words *phren*=diaphragm, mind, spirit and *logos*=word, speech, study), survived its founder for some time. In 1843 a Phrenology Journal was established in Germany. Textbooks appeared, and as late as 1863 Gall's principles were still approved by the anatomist Hermann Welcker. Most scientists, however, now disregarded his ideas.

Flourens and his doves

Considerable influence, lasting for several decades, was exerted by the work of a French physiologist, Marie Jean Pierre Flourens, in experiments with doves; he published his findings in 1824.

He removed the doves' cerebrum wholly or in part, and then carefully observed their behaviour. Doves without a cerebrum gave the impression of being completely robbed of their will-power, as if their consciousness had been extinguished. They could still move all the parts of their body, but the movements took place mechanically: they needed an impulse from outside. They walked if pushed, flew if thrown into the air, resisted if teased. They swallowed objects put into their beaks, but could not rouse themselves to eat of their own accord, even when nearly starving and there was enough food within range. Without external stimuli they sat there lost to the world as if asleep.

Flourens concluded from these results that the cerebrum was the only seat of the will and the emotions. This was no contradiction of Gall's theories. But he also carried out experiments in which he did not remove the whole brain. What he observed then led him to quite different conclusions from those drawn by Gall. If he removed only half the cerebrum, the doves retained their normal control over all bodily movements. At first they often showed a weakness in the movements of the half of the body opposite the removed half of the cerebrum. But once recovered from the operation, they were no different from normal doves with both halves of the cerebrum.

In another series of experiments Flourens removed slices of the cerebrum. On the loss of a definite amount of cerebrum, the will suddenly 'went out', and the dove sank into lethargy. But if he broke off the operation at this point, it regained the impulse apparently lost and could survive for a long time as if it had not been deprived of any of its brain substance. This recovery took place regardless of which parts of the cerebrum it had lost and which had remained intact.

Flourens's conclusion, which was shared by other experts, was that there were no organs in the cerebrum for various faculties, but that the cerebrum in its entirety was responsible for mental characteristics. It was an unexceptionable conclusion for doves; but extrapolated for the human brain, it proved a hasty and unreliable generalisation. Many scientists who rightly rejected Gall's doctrine of the brain failed to keep this distinction in mind. Isolated findings which contradicted Flourens's conclusions were for a long time paid very little attention. This was the case till 1861, when the Parisian surgeon Paul Broca established that patients with certain speech disorders regularly showed an injury to the cerebral cortex in a fixed area of the left frontal lobe. He concluded that this cortical region must house a speech centre.

Dissectors at work on the brain maps

Two scientists in Berlin, Gustav Theodor Fritsch and Eduard Hitzig, then introduced an epoch of brain research designed to discover through exact experiments what Gall had tried to find out with his unserviceable methods— all the functions of the cortex.

The starting-point of their investigations was an observation made by Fritsch as medical officer in the German–Danish war of 1864 while treating a soldier with brain damage: if places on one side of the exposed brain were stimulated with an electrical current, parts of the body on the opposite side began to twitch.

Fritsch and Hitzig systematically stimulated the cortex of dogs. As there was no suitable laboratory available in the Physiological Institute, they carried out their first studies in Hitzig's home—in fact the operations took place on Frau Hitzig's dresser. When they turned stronger currents on to precisely defined areas of the cortex, whole groups of muscles were set in motion. With weaker currents, however, they succeeded in differentiating very precisely which part of the cortex was responsible for which muscular movement.

Though the structure of a dog's brain is basically similar to that of a man's, it is not comparable in the finer details. Even the brain convolutions are different from those of a human brain. So while it might be assumed that stimulation points for muscular movements could be found on the human cortex as well, it could not be expected that they would be discovered at the equivalent places.

Once it was established that there was after all something to chart in the brain, many scientists set to work with a will. To produce a map of the human brain, results of animal experiments could point the way; but the most important information had to be gained from the human brain itself.

This had its difficulties. Inside its firmly closed skull, the live human brain is normally inaccessible to research even for harmless experiments. There was never any question of opening a healthy person's skull in quest of knowledge. To be able to help people with diseased or damaged brains, however, it is often necessary to penetrate the skull, and this provides the opportunity for learning something about the human brain. Doctors know their patients' complaints and see during the operation which areas of the brain are disturbed in their functioning by a tumour, a haemorrhage or a blood clot.

In fact we owe all discoveries about the human brain, so far as they were achieved by direct observations on live brains, to the victims of injuries and illnesses. Luckily, one can say that for the most part these patients too have benefited by the discoveries. Brain research and neurosurgery have been mutually promotive. Neither would have made any essential progress without the rapid development of the other.

In the first decades of this century, however, anatomists dominated the brain-research 'scene'. Patiently the dissection artists cut up prepared brains into tens of thousands of delicate slices—31,000 in the case of Lenin's brain, dissected in Berlin's Kaiser Wilhelm Institute for Brain Research—to study the structure of the tissue. The disciples of 'cyto-architectonics', the doctrine that the brain was a structure of cells in accordance with architectonic laws, looked especially for differences in the structure of the cortex.

In the first years of this century, after extensive anatomical studies, brain researchers believed they could draw a 'map' of the projection of functions in the cerebral cortex (on the chart above the outside of the left hemisphere is shown; below, the inside of the right hemisphere). Many apparently precise projections, however, proved questionable.

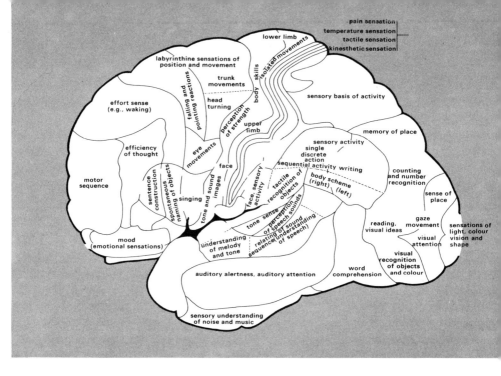

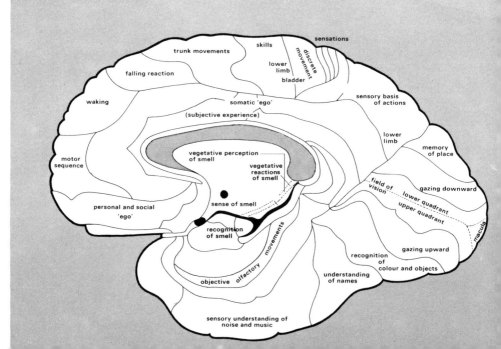

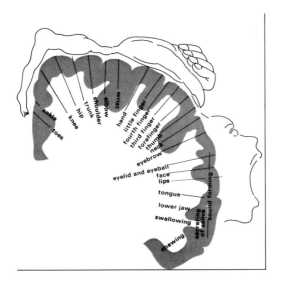

In the motor cortex in the cerebrum, by which the bodily movements are controlled, the functions are not distributed at random. In each hemisphere they can be put together into the picture of a half man. This 'cortical homunculus' is characterised by a huge hand and a big mouth.

They worked up what they found into maps of the brain embracing every small spot on the brain's surface. Eventually the brain was divided into exactly defined fields, though there were considerable differences between the maps produced. Korbinian Brodmann, for instance, believed he had seen 52 cortical fields, Cecile and Oskar Vogt about 200, Constantin von Economo 107—to name only the best-known brain anatomists of the period.

Once the fields had been discovered on anatomical criteria, they had also to be filled with significance. Many of the functions stated were uncontroversial, but others were assigned to particular fields on the basis of findings that were accidental, obscure or hard to interpret. The end products were striking brain maps which gave the impression of great exactitude, but which promised far more in the way of exact information than they could give. A few years ago the Hamburg neurologist Rudolf Janzen made the diplomatic judgement on K. Kleist's brain map reproduced here, that it 'combined the fruits and the errors of an important research tradition'.

The half man of the cortex

Brain researchers today are content with brain maps less detailed but offering far more reliable information. It is no longer a case of distinguishing dozens of sharply defined cortical fields, but a few centres with rather fluid borders which reflect knowledge about individual differences. Within the centres, at least in several, there is again division of labour. For instance, there is the motor cortex responsible for muscular movements, which Fritsch and Hitzig first systematically investigated on dogs. With men it lies in the precentral gyrus or convolution in front of the 'Rolandic fissure', which in both hemispheres runs down sideways from about the middle of the crown of the head.

This strip in each hemisphere, about an inch wide, controls the muscles with which we carry out voluntary movements. If the right place on the cortex is stimulated by electrical current, a finger moves. At other places the current makes a leg muscle twitch, the lips swell out, or causes a swallowing movement.

Stimulation of the motor cortex in the right hemisphere produces muscular movements on the left side of the body, and a corresponding cross-over effect is shown when points on the left hemisphere are stimulated. Some few muscle groups, however, such as those of the brow and the eyelids, the larynx and the tongue, and also the chewing muscles, react on both sides of the body when there is electrical stimulation in either hemisphere.

The points at which the various muscular movements can be produced by electrical stimulation are not distributed at random in the motor cortex. It is possible to map out on the motor cortex of each hemisphere the places where various body regions are represented. The resulting maps have the shape of a half man, whose foot up to the knee goes into the deep cleft which divides the two hemispheres. From the crown downwards come the other parts of the body, hip and trunk, shoulder, elbow and hand, neck and head.

But this *homunculus*, as brain researchers call the half-man picture produced by putting together the stimulation points, looks grotesque. The leg and especially the trunk are tiny compared to the hand and the head, and on the head the mouth is represented by an extremely large area of the motor cortex.

If we had not already long known it, we could read off from the cortex man's special characteristics: the hand capable of versatile movements and therefore so adroit, and the ability to utter sounds of various kinds, the precondition for differentiated linguistic understanding. In this sense the picture of *homunculus* appears more human than our actual picture. With animals the faculties in the motor cortex are differently distributed: in a pig's cortex, for instance, the snout is outsize; in a horse's, the skin round the nostrils; in a flexible and prehensile-tailed monkey's, the tail region.

Sometimes for medical reasons patients have their motor cortex stimulated. They are fully conscious, with only a local anaesthetic. What do they feel? They do not feel anything. They are all the more amazed that muscles suddenly twitch or parts of the body move unexpectedly and involuntarily. It is no good trying to resist these movements. 'Your electricity', said a patient to the physiologist José Delgado at Yale University, 'is stronger than my will.'

If parts of the motor cortex need to be removed, say during the excision of a cancerous growth, the patient also feels nothing at first. It is not till he is asked to make a movement for which the excised tissue was responsible that he discovers it doesn't work any more.

Adjacent to the motor cortex, separated from it only by the striking fissure of Rolando, lies the 'sensory cortex' in the posterior central convolution of each hemisphere. In this strip, very like the motor cortex in size and shape, the information from the mobile parts of the body comes together. It has nothing to do with feelings, say, of pain, but it receives many of the communications which form the condition for precise movement; without their continual processing, deliberate and harmonious movements cannot be made.

At each moment of the movement the position of the part of the body moved is different, and the state of the muscles changes too. The brain is in constant need of information from the muscles and joints, so that it can continually re-programme the impulses directed on the movement apparatus. Anyone who has ever tried to walk with a leg which has gone to sleep will have some idea of how necessary such a feedback is.

Brain researchers were also able to chart the sensory cortex. Electrical stimulation produced characteristic sensations in the parts of the body concerned: pricking, feelings of deafness or electricity or the impression of having made a movement when one really hadn't. The result of many stimulation experiments was again a *homunculus* on either side, very similar to that of the motor cortex.

Visual and auditory cortex

Other effects again are produced by electrical stimulation of the brain cortex at the occipital lobes. The patient imagines he is seeing flashes of light, changes of brightness or even pictures. This part, the visual cortex, processes information coming from the retina of the eye.

Stimulation of brain tissue in the furthest back corner of the occipital lobe produces only simple points of light. They do not appear at random places in the visual field. The area in which they appear depends on the stimulation point. As in the motor and sensory cortex, the various parts of the body are represented by fixed regions, so the hindmost part of the visual cortex is a projection from the retina.

Outside this central area of the visual cortex lie the 'visual association areas'. More complex perceptions occur here on electrical stimulation. The current, for instance, may produce the impression that coloured bullets are soaring into an infinite sky. The association fields have been interpreted by some as storehouses for visual information. Such storehouses are indispensable for identifying the impressions which flow in from the retina. What has just been seen is continually being compared with the stored impressions. Without this possibility the visual impressions passed on by the retina appear senseless. People whose association areas have been damaged can still see and can describe exactly the shape and colour of what they see, but they have difficulties in recognising what they have seen. It is hard to transpose oneself into the world of such a 'visually agnosic' person, as the doctors call it.

Those who are completely blind in the normally used sense, that is who no longer see anything at all, are people who have lost the retinal projections to the visual cortex through injury or illness; and they are irrevocably 'cortex blind'. No matter how sharp the eye and effective the retina, they are no good if the visual cortex is not intact. Parts of the visual field can also remain dark, depending on the extent of the cortical damage. The destruction of the whole visual cortex in one hemisphere leads to the loss of half the visual field, the left half if it is the right hemisphere, and vice versa.

As the loss of relatively small amounts of brain tissue has

such drastic effects, it seems all the more astonishing that the patient who has to have his visual cortex removed, say for a cancerous tumour, does not at first feel anything.

'As a neurosurgeon,' writes Wilder Penfield:

'I have found it necessary, as many neurosurgeons have, to remove large areas of cerebral cortex on one side from a patient while he was still conscious, using local anesthesia. As long as the brain stem is not molested, the patient remains conscious and, curiously enough, is not aware of any changes until he turns his attention to a proposition that calls for specific use of the removed portion of his cerebral cortex. Then he may discover, for example, that he cannot feel accurately what he touches with the left hand or that, although he still sees to the right, he no longer sees objects on the left.'

Comparable to cortical and mental blindness are cortical and mental deafness, which occur on loss of the 'auditory cortex'. This is a narrow strip in the top convolution of the temporal lobe. In this area, too, something characteristic happens when the tissue is stimulated by an electrical current: the patient 'hears' noises which exist only in his brain. They are never pure notes but always complex perceptions like ringing, knocking, honking, rattling, rustling or twittering; or, as patients described the noises they heard, like 'the sound of a tram passing' or 'the whistling of the wind in the trees'. When one side is stimulated, the patient has the impression that those noises are registered by both ears, but the perception seems to be stronger with the ear opposite the stimulated side.

Speech centres

This is by no means the end of the weird effects which can be produced in the cortex by a minute electrical current.

During stimulation experiments, for instance, the following can happen: while the current is flowing, the patient is shown a picture of a foot. 'What's that?' asks the experimenter. The patient cannot find the word 'foot'. He dodges. 'I know what it is. It's what you put in your shoe.' Directly the current is switched off, the word he has been hunting for is familiar to him again—'foot', he says at once. Soon afterwards he is incapable of finding the word 'tree' while the current is on. Another patient is supposed to identify a butterfly, but he says nothing. 'I couldn't think of the word "butterfly",' he reports after the current is switched off. 'Then I hunted for the word "moth", but that wouldn't come to me either.' A third patient under electrical stimulation of the brain has a comb shown to him and can say what it is used for—'I comb my hair'—but the noun 'comb' doesn't come up for him.

Such reactions are reported by Wilder Penfield in Montreal, who has provided important insights into the human brain's speech centres as well as the other parts of the 'cortical map'. His stimulation experiments, in fact, started from a wish to learn more about the speech centres for the benefit of many of his patients.

Paul Broca, it is true, had in 1861 discovered in the left frontal lobe a region to which he attributed a connection with the power of speech; but this became a subject for violent dispute among the experts. Doctors kept reporting cases of patients whose speech region (as Broca had indicated it) was destroyed, but who had no trouble in speaking. A decade later the German psychiatrist Carl Wernicke described a second speech centre which he localised in the upper part of the temporal lobe, also in the left hemisphere. But this was far from clearing up the situation. It seemed unthinkable that the variety of speech disorders called aphasia, which doctors observed in patients with intact speech organs, could be connected with a particular pattern in the cortex. There was agreement quite early on, however, that in the vast majority of mankind only the left hemisphere is concerned with speech.

The uncertainty as to which parts of the left side of the cortex were really involved in speech, led to neurosurgeons becoming scared of carrying out necessary operations in wide regions of that hemisphere. They were afraid of producing an aphasia, and refused to operate even in cases where an injury or a tumour threatened the patient's life. That side of the cortex was regarded as untouchable.

Like other neurosurgeons Penfield was constantly treating epileptics, whose complaint arose from brain damage in the forbidden area but who had no difficulties in speaking. If the position of the cortical regions really necessary for speech were successfully located, he told himself, perhaps we could operate after all in the tricky zone. He hoped that electrical brain stimulation would produce characteristic effects on the speech regions also, and that these experiments might make it possible to weigh up the advantages and dangers of an operation.

Many patients could, in fact, be helped in this way. In his investigations he marked out three speech regions. He discovered that they had varying degrees of importance for the faculty of speech (judging by how far they could be dispensed with) ; and he made a great many other interesting observations. His reports on what could be done in the brain by a minute electrical current working on a small area made it seem even harder to grasp that our brain normally functions without disturbance.

Under the electrical stimulation patients found themselves incapable of putting names to ordinary things. Besides that, the current often produced temporarily slurred or slowed-up speech, in which the words sometimes sounded distorted. In other cases the patients would say words or syllables over again. In counting they might say '6, 20, 9 . . .'. They could still distinguish, however, between numerals and other words. Sometimes, while the current was on, they mixed up words which sounded alike, such as 'camel' and 'camera', used words that didn't mean quite what they wanted, like 'shears' for 'scissors', or used totally wrong words—'place' for 'scissors' or 'brush' for 'hammer'.

Penfield could produce such disorders in three cortical regions of the left hemisphere. Two had already been found by Broca and Wernicke, but Penfield's investigations made it possible to define these regions more clearly than before. He discovered the third in the medial part (middle) of the motor cortex. Differences in the kind of disorders produced have not been substantiated, nor can the speech regions yet be subdivided into well-graded functional areas, as with the motor cortex and the visual cortex.

This has not been for want of effort. Many researchers have undertaken studies of aphasia, distinguishing various forms of such common speech disorders, in the hope of gaining a deeper insight into the speech process by working out their special features. The fruits of their labours have disappointed the experts, though for the layman many observations have been astounding enough.

Two sorts of aphasia

Neurologists distinguish two main forms of speech disorders (other than those caused by inadequate functioning of the speech organs): motor and sensory aphasia. With the former, the patient understands everything said to him, but cannot put into the right words what he has to communicate. With the latter the patient can speak, though what he says often sounds rather nonsensical, but he does not understand what is said to him. A word he may just have uttered himself is completely incomprehensible to him, and this is not because of bad hearing.

With slighter cases of motor aphasia, patients show similar symptoms to those of Penfield's patients on electrical stimulation of a speech region. But their powers of speech are often much more seriously disturbed, so that as a rule they cannot read or write either. Clearly, they lack the capacity for representing thoughts symbolically, the pre-condition for people to understand each other. Even sign language, normally a last resort in communication difficulties, ceases to function—which is a terrible loss, of course, to any deaf-mutes suffering from aphasia. Aphasics often cannot even nod their heads for 'yes' and shake it for 'no': the gestures, which are also symbols of conceptual thinking, are lost with the words. The difficulties which aphasics have to overcome in forming concepts can even be recognised in the wax models made by patients of Eberhard Bay at the Neurological Clinic, Dusseldorf University: an egg is not an egg but a ball, a pot is like a plate; and a figure described by its aphasic creator as 'bird or ship' shows a strange hybrid, half duck, half fish.

Aphasics are sometimes surprisingly good at using stereotyped phrases and they have little difficulty with swearing and cursing. One of the cases brought forward at the end of the last century as an argument against the existence of a specialised speech centre was a patient at the Munich Asylum, who after an apoplectic fit was conspicuous for his continual loud swearing. When he had died, the doctors found the region given by Broca as a speech centre completely destroyed. This discovery made the Munich psychiatrist Bernhard von Gudden a bitter opponent of those who considered the existence of a speech centre as proved. The contradiction is resolved, however, when one remembers that the problem facing aphasics is the difficulty of forming concepts. Swearwords, like stereo-type phrases, contain no information, require no process of concept-forming. 'The oath', writes Eberhard Bay, 'does not belong at all in the actual realm of human language, but in pre-linguistic communication. It is on a level with the growling and barking of an angry animal. Man expresses his discontent in articulate speech only because that is as familiar to him as barking to a dog.'

A swearing aphasic is sometimes incapable of repeating, when asked, the oath he has just uttered. Or, if you say the word 'no' to an aphasic and tell him to repeat it, he may be unable to manage it—and eventually say resignedly: 'No, I can't do it', not realising that he has said the word he was looking for.

This is all very hard to understand for anyone hearing about it for the first time. The physical conditions for speaking are there, and so are words, even if they are often the wrong ones or meaningless. Sometimes an aphasic even puts in the right word, but it comes in unconsciously and out of context. Is the disturbed relation of aphasics to speech caused perhaps by impaired intelligence? The idea sounds plausible, but it does not work out. Apart from their speech difficulties, including the weakness in reading and writing, they behave quite normally. With practical intelligence unimpaired, they do not stand out as odd until they have to speak.

The Soviet neuropsychologist A. R. Luria of Moscow University has reported the case of a famous patient suffering from sensory aphasia—that is, unable to understand speech any more—who enhanced his fame in unimpaired creativity. This was the composer Vissarion Shebalin: robbed of his understanding of speech by a haemorrhage in the left temporal lobe, he continued, says Luria, 'to create wonderful symphonies'.

It all sounds amazing, almost incredible. But the striking phenomena of aphasia are all produced by the same laws, so far too little known, by which our own brains function.

Filmstrip experiences

In his studies of the left hemisphere, extending over

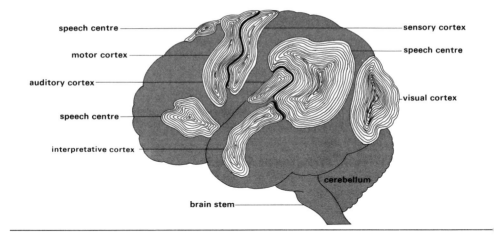

This is what the modern map of the outside of the left cerebral hemisphere looks like. In contrast to the details on the old maps, the particulars seem well confirmed.

decades, Penfield became convinced that the two frontal speech regions were to some extent dispensable without causing lasting damage, but that extensive injury to the great posterior speech region gave little hope of the aphasia being removed.

The easiest to replace is the speech region at the motor cortex. Even when it is completely destroyed, this leads to only temporary speech difficulties: the aphasia disappears within a few weeks. The region in the lower part of the frontal lobe seems less easy to replace, but Penfield came across patients in whom this region was destroyed and who nevertheless spoke quite normally. The destroyed tissue, however, had led to epileptic fits. The past history of these patients showed that they had received head wounds years before and that their powers of speech, destroyed thereby, had gradually come back. Obviously other areas of the cortex could take over the functions of this speech centre. To eliminate the seat of the epileptic fits, Penfield cut out the destroyed tissue, without provoking any speech disorders by so doing.

He could not find out which were the areas that took over the function of the destroyed speech region. He found no support for the idea that the right hemisphere 'leapt into the breach'. Electrical stimulation there did not lead to the symptoms of aphasia, as observed with the left hemisphere. But his investigations were not systematically pursued, since patients are not guinea-pigs.

Soon after the beginning of his stimulation experiments to define the speech regions, Penfield produced with the electrical probe the first filmstrip experiences. They could be provoked in both hemispheres. Optical scenes ran predominantly in the 'inarticulate' right hemisphere, while acoustic and combined experiences were rather more frequent in the left.

All the illusory impressions were produced in the temporal lobes: in the left hemisphere, only outside the great speech region; in the right, in wider areas. The cortical areas which presented such reactions Penfield called 'interpretative cortex', on the hypothesis that this area of the cortex helped us to order our experiences by comparing them with earlier ones. 'It is apparent,' he writes, 'that in any normal individual, when the present experience resembles strikingly an experience from the past, that past is summoned reflexly, automatically. A man is not aware of the summoning until the interpretation, for example, that the situation is familiar or dangerous, flashes up in consciousness. Presently, the subject discovers that the data from the past has come within voluntary reach. The man, or the place, you saw last perhaps 15 years ago, comes back to you sufficiently so you can check off the changes which time has wrought in him, or in it.'

For the time being this is still theory. It is also not clear yet where the filmstrips are stored. Penfield does not believe that the 'film archives' are in the temporal lobes where the illusions are produced. When a cortical area which had provided a filmstrip experience had to be removed, the memory of the illusion was by no means wiped out.

A considerable part of the cortex is filled out with motor and sensory cortex, visual and auditory cortex, speech regions and interpretative cortex. But there are still white patches on the map of the fissured brain surface, places where the 'explorers' cannot yet speak with any confidence. The great white patch in the front part of the frontal lobe is not really white. This part of the cortex has a special relationship with intention and purpose.

6

Surgery for the Psyche?

On 13 September 1848 Phineas Gage, a foreman in the
construction of an American railway line, did what he had
often done before; he prepared for a blasting operation.
Powder had already been poured into the borehole, and it
should actually have been covered over with sand; but this
was not done. When Gage thrust a tamping-iron into the
borehole as usual, the charge exploded.

The pointed iron shaft, some three and a half feet long
and over an inch thick, shot through his head. It entered at
the left cheek, coming diagonally from below, penetrated
the brain in the region of the frontal lobe, and flew up and
out through the skull. Did this mean instant death? Not
at all. He fell on his back, but remained conscious. Workmen
carried him several miles to the road. He sat up in the oxcart
which took him home, climbed out of the cart without
much help, and went up a long flight of stairs. 'The iron',
he told the doctor, pointing to the wound, 'went in there
and right through my head.'

He recovered, and those who met him casually did not
notice any effects of the severe injury he had suffered. No
part of his body let him down, he remained fully responsible

for his actions, his memory functioned as before the accident. He periodically earned a livelihood by exhibiting himself and the tamping-iron. Twelve years after the accident he died in San Francisco—not of his brain injury. His pierced skull and the tamping-iron are still on show today at Harvard's Warren Museum.

His contemporaries were amazed not only that he survived the accident but that the severe damage undoubtedly borne by his brain seemed to affect him so little. It seems surprising to us, too. If the destruction of small parts in the area of the motor cortex, the visual cortex or the speech regions, produces serious disorders, paralysing parts of the body, obscuring whole areas of the visual field, drastically restricting powers of expression and speech—one would expect such an immense loss of brain tissue as Gage suffered to have had far more striking effects.

It sounds all the more probable because a comparison of human and animal brains shows that man is distinguished from his nearest relatives in the animal kingdom, not to mention the more distant ones, by the massive development of the cerebrum and of the frontal lobe in particular, which developed even more strongly than the whole cerebrum.

This lobe comprises about a third of the whole human cortex. With chimpanzees it is only a fifth, and a great deal less than that with less closely related animals like cats and dogs. That there must be something special about the brain directly behind man's brow was intuitively grasped by the sculptors of ancient Greece: for their gods and heroes they carved heads with a brow much higher and wider than is usually the case with normal people. It is hard to grasp that what lies behind the 'egghead' brow can easily be dispensed with.

Was the surprisingly good recovery of Phineas Gage an isolated case, then, bordering on the miraculous? Far from it. In 1870 the Berlin brain researchers Fritsch and Hitzig, the first to carry out experiments with electrical stimulation of the cortex, were already talking of 'observations in plentiful number on surgical injuries to the brain without disturbance of any functions'. Hitzig reported one such case which he had seen himself in the Berlin garrison hospital in 1866: a shell splinter had penetrated a soldier's brain between the eyebrows and torn a triangular hole there. 'Unceasing brain substance' drained from this hole for over a fortnight. Eventually the wound healed on its own, and Hitzig found that the patient showed no signs of gross motor or sensory disorders. He noted, however, that the man seemed dull-witted, although, not having known him before, Hitzig could not say whether this was natural to him or due to the injury.

People who had known Phineas Gage well before his accident did not think he had survived the brain injury unchanged. Before it, friends said, he was able and energetic, a man of careful and balanced disposition. But after his physical recovery he showed traits they had not known in him. He was now moody, obstinate and impatient, had little consideration for others and sometimes behaved (his doctor reported) with great impropriety, which was not his way before. And whereas before he had been accustomed as foreman to acting with resolution, he now found it difficult to make decisions.

For a long time such observations were not paid much attention, and when brain researchers remembered them they did not see any good starting-points for experimental investigations. If a certain area of the motor cortex were stimulated, certain muscles would twitch—one could rely on that. If a certain region of the visual cortex were destroyed in an animal, an exactly circumscribed part of the visual field would be lost. But in the front parts of the brain electrical current produced no dramatic effects whatever; and if parts of an animal's frontal lobe were cut out, the animal seemed little affected. So the frontal lobe became thought of as a 'silent' or mystery region.

To be precise, not the whole frontal lobe, for in the posterior part it has the motor cortex and two of the speech regions. The rôle of the motor cortex and one of the speech regions was recognised early, but scientists who carried out tests on the usual laboratory animals, in an attempt to discover the rôle of the prefrontal cortex—the fore-brain—made no real progress. This is not surprising, since as we know today the fore-brain has not only developed very greatly in man but in function as well is the most distinctively 'human' part of the brain. It was experiments on chimpanzees, man's nearest relatives, in the early thirties which first brought instructive results.

If the researchers removed the fore-brain on one side, there were scarcely any effects to be observed; but without the whole of it the chimpanzees proved no longer up to complex tasks. They were incapable of solving a problem which consisted of three successive actions. Similar impairments had been observed in men with fore-brain injuries: these patients often found it hard to keep several thoughts in their head at a time and to bring them to a rational conclusion.

One of the observations made on chimpanzees gave the impulse for the first 'psychosurgical' brain operations, in which the surgeons deliberately tried to achieve some psychological changes and accepted others as inevitable side-effects of hoped-for favourable results.

When chimpanzees were set problems too hard for them, which they therefore could not solve at all, and this happened several times in succession, they became furious, yelling and screaming, rattling at the cage bars, and rolling about on the ground. If the problems set them proved insoluble over a longer period, they retired into a corner of the cage, refused to eat anything and could not be used for any further experiments. If, however, their frontal lobes were removed, this abnormal behaviour disappeared. They were once more as friendly and co-operative as ever. Outbursts of rage stopped at once. Admittedly they made many more mistakes than before the operation; but this no longer upset them.

Leucotomy becomes fashionable

These results were described by the American psychologist Carlyle Jacobsen of Yale at the International Neurological Congress in London in 1935. His audience included a remarkable man of sixty-one who was Professor of Neurology at Lisbon University: to give him his full name, Antonio Caetano de Abreu Freire Egas Moniz. At twenty-nine Egas Moniz had become a Portuguese member of parliament, at thirty-seven director of the newly established Neurological Institute at Lisbon University. He was for a time Portuguese Ambassador in Madrid, and as foreign minister led his country's delegation to the Paris Peace Conference in 1919. In the medical world he had achieved a world-wide reputation by introducing 'cerebral angiography', a process enabling the brain's blood vessels to be made visible on X-rays.

Hearing Jacobsen's findings, Egas Moniz was very much impressed by the change of personality which the operations had produced on the chimpanzees. He thought of some of his seriously disturbed patients, suffering from uncontrollable anxiety and aggressiveness, and felt that such an operation would mean an improvement for them. He had been working on this before as well. Seeing Jacobsen and learning about his results gave him a fillip. Returning to Lisbon, he acted on these ideas, and the same year operated on his first patients with the neurosurgeon Almeida Lima as colleague. They did not cut out the whole fore-brain, hoping to achieve the same effects with a more limited operation.

They introduced into the patient's brain a cannula (long

needle) with a small blade about a fifth of an inch long stuck into its point. When the needle reached the right place, they made the blade snap open, and by turning the needle cut through many of the white nerve fibres leading from the fore-brain cortex to the inner regions of the brain. Then the blade was shut and the needle withdrawn. The procedure was repeated at three to five other places in the fore-brain.

In 1936 Egas Moniz reported on the first twenty patients who had been operated on in Lisbon. Seven were 'cured' and seven 'improved'; with the other six there was no change. What is meant by the words in quotation marks? Patients who before the operation were inclined to fits of rage and dangerously impulsive actions, who suffered from tormenting fear and heightened irritability, continual anxiety and insomnia or suicidal tendencies, seemed calmer. The urge to violence had disappeared. Emotional tensions had abated.

But these improvements had to be paid for. The patients operated on showed similar personality changes to others with brain damage. Their calm could better be called indifference. They often spent the rest of their days in dull apathy without initiative or any real interest in life. If they had had any ambition, it had gone, and they had little sense of responsibility. If they had any creative abilities, those too had been extinguished.

Considering, however, that Egas Moniz and Lima had operated only on patients with the most severe psychological disorders, it is understandable that many doctors all over the world were more strongly impressed by the operation's positive effects than by the risks involved. Leucotomies, so called because white brain substance was cut through (from the Greek *leukos* = white and *tomé* = cut), spread widely in the forties, and with various new methods developed into the standard brain operation in more and more theatres, especially in the United States. As Hans Heimann of Berne University's Psychiatric Clinic wrote in 1963 in his textbook

Psychiatrie der Gegenwart (Psychology of the Present), 'very soon surgery was carried out for all possible conditions and complaints, and psychosurgery became the therapeutic craze'. This happened, said Heimann, 'without any secure theoretical basis or clear indication principles, under the influence of the hopelessness of many psychiatric illnesses and many patients who seemed doomed to a wretched asylum life.'

Because it was the fashion, many patients had the operation where the indications were dubious from the out-set. Alcoholics, for instance, justifiably worried about their future, were given leucotomies on request; afterwards they went on drinking but were no longer worried about it. There was criticism on other counts too: enthusiasts for leucotomy were confronted by passionate objectors to the whole idea.

The latter argued that it was directed against man's highest mental and spiritual faculties, closely bound up with the individual personality, that it was a thorough mental and spiritual mutilation, and was carried out on people who were often not in a position to recognise its magnitude: it was, in fact, a unique attack on personal integrity. This factor was accepted by authorities who refused to be dogmatically for or against the operation, believing that in every case the possible benefits should be strictly balanced against the risks: with scrupulous examina-tion one might then decide that it was better for the patient to go on living with an altered personality but less acute agony than to continue in his old condition without prospect of improvement.

In 1948 the first International Congress for Psychosurgery took place in Lisbon. Egas Moniz, who was awarded the Nobel Prize for medicine the following year, was not present to defend his 'baby'. But in the years after that, neurosurgeons leucotomised thousands of patients a year. By 1954 up to 50,000 leucotomies had been performed in the United States, about 10,000 in Britain. The numbers were very much smaller in Germany; and in Russia the operation was banned in 1950—on ideological grounds rather than out of concern for the patients. Pavlov and Bechterev, recognised as the authorities on brain research, had stated decades earlier that psychological disorders involved the whole brain and not particular regions of it; they could not therefore be improved by operations on such regions.

The new fashion had already passed its peak. The year 1952 saw the discovery of the first psychoactive drugs with which doctors could effectively treat abnormal psychological conditions. Within a few years there was a drastic change in the world's psychiatric clinics and mental hospitals. Though these drugs too, have their problems, even confirmed supporters of leucotomy now preferred to use drugs in most cases where they had formerly operated. Leucotomy today is confined to relatively few cases where nothing else helps. In certain rare circumstances, for instance, it may be considered for patients with schizophrenia, with severe compulsion neuroses resistant to treatment, for old people with chronic depressions, mentally deficient people who are constantly aggressive and patients with pain that cannot be alleviated, especially in the head. The pain does not disappear, but after the operation they do not make anything of it: their unpleasant emotional reaction to pain has changed, not the actual sensation.

The dangers of psychosurgery

Psychosurgery revealed for the first time in full sharpness the double edge of brain research, with benefit and risk lying closer together than in any other sphere. Moreover, several researchers and surgeons, fascinated by the possibility of manipulating their patients' brains, overstepped the bounds of their responsibility. Happily, this development did not escalate but soon died down; and it is perhaps some consolation to the families of patients leucotomised without urgent reasons that the patients themselves did not mind afterwards, this being one of the operation's after-effects.

The observations on thousands of patients who had the connection between the fore-brain cortex and the control centres more or less drastically broken off, provided a detailed picture of the influence exerted on the human mind by the fore-brain cortex. The behaviour of leucotomised patients reveals what the lack of a fore-brain cortex means for a person. Hans Heimann has described typical features:

'The leucotomised man shows the picture of a personality in decline. Physically he looks robust to heavy. In his movements and his reasoning he is slow and often rather fussy. He is a late riser, goes to bed early, likes a comfortable life and plenty of good food. He takes a passive attitude to the problems of life, chooses the line of least resistance and is generally carefree. This is accompanied by a generally cheerful to euphoric outlook, impaired powers of self-criticism, specially in regard to his own abilities, an avoidance of responsibility and reduced sense of obligation. It is always noticeable that he fails to grasp more complicated situations, and that although relatively inconspicuous in his usual environment he cannot face unexpected new problems. He makes no plans for the future, doesn't bother much altogether about what lies ahead for him, just as he forgets about the past and is absorbed like a child in the present. . . . Although there is no temporal disorientation in the strict sense—the primitive sense and awareness of time are undisturbed—he has lost his relationship with being "in time".

'Taken up with the present, he is also more dependent on excitement, can be influenced and distracted by everything which directly impinges on him. In company he lets himself be carried along passively, without taking the lead in a conversation himself. His contributions are meagre, unoriginal and severely limited by his condition with its attention to trivia and its claims to food and comfort. He does not make any real contact with the person he is talking to, is insensitive to finer feelings, and therefore often chatters away tactlessly, makes stupid jokes at which he laughs loudly himself, showing that he is out of touch with the atmosphere of his company. He is extremely self-centred; and this, especially in the family circle, makes him vent his moods and tempers on its members. He may fall into tantrums of childish obstinacy and petulance, but has no consideration for the objections and claims of the others.

'He is without pride, shame or regret, and is characterised by the shallowness of his emotions and personality generally. His interests are directed on superficial conversation and immediate satisfaction of appetites, without higher claims or creative qualities. It is often observed that religious interests and conflicts which existed before have disappeared. ... In short, his experience horizon has narrowed and flattened out.'

Although the 'average' leucotomised patient is something like this, there are marked variations in the extent of the charactistics. No satisfactory explanation has yet been found, for instance, as to why loss of drive and inhibitions occur more in one patient than another. The most puzzling of all are the few patients among thousands who, after a leucotomy, not only could cope with relatively undemanding activities, but were capable of working again in independent and responsible positions. One played in a first-class symphony orchestra, another went out to Africa as a missionary, a third worked as a registrar in a mental hospital, a fourth obtained a responsible post in the civil service. Unless one supposed that when operating the doctors failed to cut through the nerve fibres, the only possibility left seems to be that these brains found ways of compensating for injuries which normally lead to severe stunting of mind and personality. A lot depends, of course, on the area and extent of the prefrontal damage.

Considering the changes produced as a rule by the neuro-surgeon's sensitive hand through small deliberate cuts in the brain of the leucotomised patient, it is not surprising that severe injuries to the fore-brain in wars and after accidents often have equally drastic consequences—as was the case indeed with Phineas Gage on closer inspection. These patients also lose initiative, find it hard to act purposefully and think rationally, but such disorders may be manifested in still higher degree.

Many victims of fore-brain injuries, when called on to do something, instead of consistent actions to that end, will often merely carry out endless repetitions of the first step. There are reports of a man who tried to light a match that was burning, of another planing clean through a board when he wanted to polish its surface and then going on to plane the hotel bench underneath.

Alexander Luria, Director of the Neuropsychological Department of Moscow University, who for decades has made extensive examinations of thousands of brain-damaged patients, reports on a woman with damage to the fore-brain, who wrote to a colleague of his, 'Dear Professor, I would like to say to you that I would like to say to you that I would like to say to you . . .' and so on, for pages. Other patients, if they had to tell a story, could not get past the first sentence. They found it hard to order their thoughts and concentrate on an aim. They complained of not remembering anything, that they needed hours or days, for instance, to write a simple letter, which then never got beyond 'Dear X, many thanks for your letter'.

Luria also reported that fore-brain-damaged patients made very peculiar interpretations of easily recognisable pictures. A deathbed scene was regarded as a wedding— because of the solemn clothes, the patient said; a mourner drying her tears with a handkerchief was thought to have a cold. Obviously the ability to connect the individual data into a rational whole has been destroyed.

Investigations initiated by such observations showed the difficulty such patients found in looking at any picture normally. Luria registered their eye movements when they were looking at one. The pattern was fundamentally different from the eye movement pattern of ordinary people, who look at a picture systematically and, if asked questions about it, direct their attention to characteristic details; the eyes of those with fore-brain damage wander over the picture at random.

Neither observations on leucotomised patients nor on those with fore-brain damage have given any indications that particular areas of the fore-brain cortex represent special psychological components, in the way that the visual cortex does for the various regions of the visual field or the motor cortex for the individual parts of the body. Clearly, there is no psychological mosaic on the fore-brain cortex; apparently the fore-brain carries out its important functions as a whole, which means that injuries of varying extent and kinds may be compensated for.

The brain surface, which looks so unified despite convolutions, really consists of various organs. Is there an order there? Luria divides the cerebral cortex into two 'blocks', one formed by the frontal lobes, the other by the temporal, parietal and occipital lobes. While the rear block plays the decisive rôle in processing information, analysing, interpreting and storing it when it comes in, the front block is occupied with fixing and following aims as well as working out a behaviour programme.

'*Cogito, ergo sum.*' Over three hundred years ago René Descartes made his proud statement the starting-point of his mechanistic philosophy. It seems as if it were above all the frontal lobes which gave him the possibility of producing such a statement.

7

Feelings to Order

For a fortnight José Delgado and his colleagues at Yale sat in front of a monkey's cage. The monkey was doing the same thing over and over again exactly once a minute, over twenty thousand times during the fortnight. Once a minute it would suddenly break off whatever other activity it was occupied with, in order to carry out a precisely fixed series of actions.

It turned right, got on to its hind-legs and walked upright a few steps round the cage. Then it climbed up a grating wall but at once came back to the ground. It uttered one or two sounds, stood on all fours and assumed a threatening posture —opening its mouth, laying back its ears, raising its tail and looking balefully across at another particular monkey in the cage. The stereotyped course of actions ended as suddenly as it had begun, and the monkey resumed the activity interrupted a few seconds before.

The animal had no neurotic tic! What it did was due to an invisible external compulsion imposed on it by the researchers outside the cage: their remote control produced this strange recurring behaviour.

Similar uncanny experiments are carried out today in

many laboratories all over the world. Researchers make animals go to sleep and wake up as required, they influence feeding and sexual drive, produce fear or rage where there is not the slightest cause for such reactions. They can create in animals such irresistible feelings of pleasure that the creatures forget everything else and would starve for pleasure if the researchers let them.

As with stimulation of the cortex, it is again electrical current which forces the brain into involuntary actions or to impressions completely unmotivated by external circumstances. The reactions mentioned, however, are produced by electrical stimuli not in the brain's outer zones but deep in the interior. By fine, stainless steel wires sunk into the brain, the current reaches stimulation places which have even more impressive effects than those on the cerebral cortex, so that animals and also men can be made into puppets of the researchers.

Thousands of people have carried and still carry electrodes in their head; and there is no doubt at all that these brain stimulations are useful for the diagnosis and treatment of illnesses. Understandably, however, few brain operations have given rise to so many speculations about a grim future, in which dictators have remote control over a subject population through electrodes planted in the brain; the switch is thrown to produce an industrious mood, with rewards and punishments, also by switch, through stimulation of a pleasure centre or production of pain.

All the attempts at external control of animal and human behaviour through electrical stimulation of the brain go back to research which the Swiss physiologist Walter Rudolf Hess started in 1924 and carried on over many years. In 1949 he was awarded—with Egas Moniz—the Nobel Prize for medicine.

He bored small holes into the skulls of anaesthetised cats and then introduced into their brains fine wires fixed into the cranial openings with the help of a plug; these served as electrodes , but they were insulated. Only at the uninsulated tips of the electrodes could current transmitted from outside act on the surrounding brain tissue. In this way Hess succeeded in producing purposeful electrical stimulation of a tiny area of the brain.

There were fears that the introduction of wires would cause serious damage to the penetrated brain tissue, but they proved groundless. Although nerve tissue was destroyed by the electrodes, the brain evidently had a built-in security system: it seemed that no single function was the responsibility of only one particular small group of nerve cells. At any rate the insertion of the electrodes produced no disorders, even when later with animals—and also with men—dozens of wires were sunk into the brain simultaneously. The electrodes can stay in their place for months or even years. They end in a kind of wall-socket which is fixed to the skull. When a certain point of the brain is to be stimulated, current only has to be transmitted by the wall-socket into the appropriate electrode.

With his electrical probes Hess palpated structures deep in the brain's interior point by point. He investigated particularly the diencephalon, which lies between brain stem and cerebrum, and observed peculiar reactions according to which area he put under the current. The cats began to eat or to lick their skin; they fell into rage or fear, without any external cause; they purred and wanted to be stroked or went to sleep under the brain stimulation.

Each of these and other kinds of behaviour could be produced at various points, some lying close together, others dispersed over a wider area. The electrical stimulus acted like an irresistible command. When an 'eating point' was stimulated, a cat would begin to eat again, even if it had just finished eating its fill. The electrically produced greed was sometimes so great that if there was nothing else available it would sometimes try to eat inedible objects.

Stimulation of other points produced in the cat a threatening posture. Whether the cat then went on to attack, confined itself to showing defensiveness, or ran away, depended on the situation. From this adaptive behaviour Hess concluded that the cats were not reacting like automata, but that the current transmitted the experience of a threat and in fact put them in an irritable mood.

Many of Hess's colleagues could not imagine electrical current penetrating so deep into the psychological condition as to elicit real emotions. They gave electricity credit merely for producing the behavioural consequences of feelings and moods, not the feelings and moods themselves. For instance, they called electrically provoked rage 'pseudo-rage'. At the time, moreover, few scientists were much interested in the new possibility of investigating the intact living brain.

This changed at the beginning of the 'fifties. Then scientists began systematically studying the brains of various creatures with electrodes. They confirmed what Hess had found on cats, and made a great many new observations both fascinating and frightening. One of the first series of experiments immediately shook the scepticism of those who could not grasp the possibility of electric current influencing psychology.

In 1953 at McGill University, Montreal, James Olds noted that a rat which had had an electrode inserted into its brain kept on going to a particular corner of the cage. It was not just any corner; directly the rat turned up there, Olds closed the circuit and transmitted some electricity into its brain. Obviously it liked the brain stimulation. The electrode must have hit a region of the brain the stimulation of which produced pleasant sensations.

To confirm this beyond doubt Olds and his colleague Peter Milner constructed a do-it-yourself device for their rats. They brought into the cage a lever which a rat could easily press down with its front paw. As soon as it did so, a circuit closed for a moment, and stimulating current flowed through the electrode into the rat's brain.

What happened then seems incredible. The rats pressed the lever up to five thousand times an hour, more than once a second, and continued to do so until they collapsed exhausted. When the current was switched off, they showed no special interest in the 'pleasure lever'. After this result no one could assert any longer that current produced only pseudo-pleasure in animals. Olds and Milner discovered a whole series of 'pleasure centres' which the rats enjoyed having stimulated. They were all deep in the brain's interior, but scattered over different structures.

With the self-stimulation device the researchers also succeeded without great difficulty in measuring the degrees of pleasure produced by the electrical stimulation at the various points: according to the electrode's position, the rats showed varying degrees of keenness to press the lever. On stimulation of some points they were content with a few hundred shocks an hour, which left them enough time for other activity. Other points provided such an irresistible feeling that they hammered on the lever tirelessly at the speed of Morse and brought it up to seven thousand shocks an hour.

To acquire the pleasure-giving shocks, the rats would pay a high price, eagerly climbing over obstacles, putting up with pain stimuli and going without food. Olds and Milner made rats used to brain stimuli fast for a day, and then put them into a cage which gave them the alternatives of current into the brain or food. They refused to eat, preferring to devote themselves continuously to self-stimulation. They never got tired of the brain stimuli.

Olds succeeded in distinguishing the electrically produced feelings of pleasure in their quality as well as their intensity. At some points the rats liked stimulating themselves more when they were hungry than when they had just eaten their fill. Apparently stimulation at these points produced the pleasant feeling of repletion. Other points revealed clearly a relation to sex: in these cases castrated young rats did not show any interest in the stimulation lever until injected with male sex hormones.

Pleasure centres in the brain are no speciality of rats. Dogs and cats, goldfish and dolphins can be fascinated by correctly placed brain stimuli, and so can monkeys and men. The psychiatrist Robert G. Heath of Tulane University, New Orleans, was the first to equip patients with pleasure-giving electrodes, and put into their hands a button with which they could switch on the current themselves. They pressed it eagerly, and when Heath asked them why they were doing so, they said the button made them happy, it gave them such a good feeling. They too went on revelling in the good feeling, often to the point of exhaustion.

As early as 1963 Heath reported that brain electrodes helped a patient to win an otherwise hopeless battle against sleep. The patient, a man of twenty-eight, suffered from narcolepsy, an illness in which people are overcome by irresistible drowsiness several times a day. Directly he felt slumber approaching, the man could press a button to transmit current into the electrode, and so himself produced a brain stimulus which banished the sleep that threatened him.

The same year as Olds in Montreal began tracking down the pleasure centres in the brain, American researchers at Yale discovered brain centres the stimulation of which was not experienced by animals as pleasurable, but clearly as extremely unpleasant. When stimulated at such points, they reacted as if tormented by violent fear or pain. A burst of current transmitted into one of these aversion centres can in a moment completely transform a monkey till then quite content with itself and the world. It makes grimaces, screams and tries to run away, shakes and shivers, its hair stands on end, its pupils are enlarged. Physically, nothing different has happened from what happens when a pleasure centre is stimulated—a small amount of current flows into the brain. Astonishingly enough, the pleasure and aversion centres are sometimes only fractions of an inch apart—but what a difference for the animal which of them is stimulated!

By stimulating specific points in animal brains, researchers have been able to produce a great many different reactions. In the Max Planck Institute for Behavioural Physiology at Seewiesen (Bavaria), Erich von Holst and Ursula von Saint Paul planted electrodes into the brains of cocks and hens. For years the birds happily ran around with the wires in their heads and could at any time demonstrate the power of a brain stimulus. Electrical stimulation was either direct or mediated by a radio control. At a radio signal a hen might begin to clean its feathers, sharpen its beak or ruffle its plumage against a non-existent enemy. The researchers reported 'that nearly all the familiar movements serving orientation and bodily needs, or relating to enemies, rivals, mates and offspring, can be activated from the brain stem with all the appropriate calls.'

Animals which have had a whole series of electrodes planted in their brains behave, said Delgado at Yale, 'like electrical toys'. Quite different reactions can be produced according to which button the experimenter presses. The complicated course of actions repeated twenty thousand times by the monkey mentioned at the beginning of this chapter was controlled by a single electrode which stimulated a specific point in the brain stem. A second electrode, its tip only an eighth of an inch away from the stimulation point of the first, scarcely had any effect. The monkey only yawned. Similar extremely specific effects have been found in man, too, and suggest terrifying possibilities for the manipulation of human beings by a ruthless dictator.

8

The Brain's Interior

The cerebrum takes up about eighty per cent of the human brain. Of the remaining twenty, half goes to the cerebellum, a sort of calculating machine for control of movements. The other ten per cent is divided between brain stem and diencephalon.

After the findings described in the last chapter, no one is likely to conclude, from the small area of the last two sectors compared with the whole human brain, that they are of minor significance. Within these sectors deep inside the head there is spontaneous regulation of many physical processes important to life, to which we normally do not pay any attention or which are altogether removed from conscious control. One of the original places responsible for feelings and emotions is also situated there, although parts of the cerebrum lying near the brain stem and diencephalon also have such functions.

For a closer look at the parts of the brain hidden under the convolutions of the cerebral cortex, we may start with the brain stem, which represents a prolongation of the spinal cord. Its position has been compared with the stalk of a flower, around which the other parts of our brain are grouped

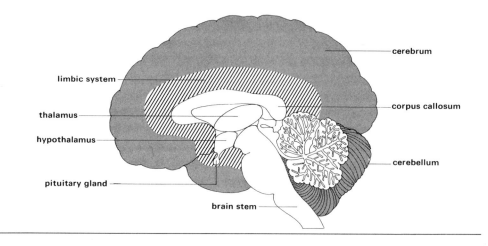

The oldest parts of the brain lie deep inside the head. Bodily functions important for life are automatically regulated there, and it is also where feelings and emotions originate.

like petals. In its deepest region it houses a system of the greatest importance for our life, the breathing centre. It automatically controls the rate and depth of respirations. It is of course obedient to impulses from the cerebrum—we can at will breathe faster or slower, deeper or shallower. But when we are not attending to our breathing, as is usually the case, the breathing centre takes over control. It reacts, however, to variations in the carbon dioxide content of the blood: if the blood contains little carbon dioxide, the breathing centre stimulates chest muscles and diaphragm to normal breathing movements; if the amount rises, breathing is speeded up.

Other centres in the brain stem regulate heart activity and blood pressure and also functions of the gastro-intestinal tract. The brain stem has functions, besides, in supervising the production of saliva and the secretion of lachrymal fluid. In it many reflexes are produced, like coughing, sneezing, vomiting; and it is the source of emotions too—containing pleasure centres the electrical stimulation of which produces the maximum of pleasure in laboratory animals.

In addition to all this, according to a disputed theory, the brain stem contains a sort of 'top management' for the whole organism. Such a system, which the brain no doubt needs, is supposed to be a striking network of nerve cells known for decades to anatomists as the reticular formation. Reassessment of this began with an Italian and an American researcher, Giuseppe Moruzzi and Horace Magoun. In 1949 they put forward the theory that it had the task of keeping the brain awake and activating it. They called the ascending part of the network the reticular activation system. Exactly how and to what extent it controls consciousness is still far from being fully understood. But at any rate the hypothesis activated the brains of many other researchers!

They found it significant that the alleged activation centre was situated at a place at which all communications must pass from the brain into the body and from the body into the brain. The network's strategically favourable position offered attractive grounds for building out of the hypothesis of cerebral activation the idea that the reticular activation system was the brain's programme selection centre where decisions were made about the priorities of particular forms of behaviour.

The management function which may be occupied by the reticular activation system is described thus by Madge E. and Arnold B. Scheibel at the University of California in Los Angeles:

'Competition for the interest of the reticular arrays must be high, and supremacy is gained for the moment in time only by those data that are most "exotic"—or most compelling biologically. Like some stern, harried father figure, the core has limited patience and limited time-binding resources; its logic is wide but superficial, its decisionary apparatus does not permit the luxury of hesitation.'

We tend to take for granted the generally practical reactions of our body and mind. But when we think about them, it seems obvious that there must be a 'court of first instance' in the brain which makes decisions from moment to moment on what we do, and which things we turn our attention to—for there would always be the possibility of doing or attending to something else. The reticular activation system might be such a first court.

Controllers for the brain's interior

The diencephalon above the brain stem consists of two parts, thalamus and hypothalamus, the latter being the lower part. It does not, however, lie right under the thalamus but protrudes a bit in front. Thalamus and hypothalamus, unlike the brain stem, are duplicated organs with one in each hemisphere. They have very different functions to fulfil. While the thalamus (generally used in the singular, although there are two organs) is in close contact with the cerebrum, the hypothalamus controls the body's internal conditions, assuring, for instance, a constant body temperature, regulating water input and output and food intake, and influencing the interplay of the hormonal glands. Electrodes placed in various parts of it can also produce many emotional reactions.

Our body temperature is normally about 98.4°F (36.5°C), and our physical well-being depends on its varying only within very narrow limits, regardless of the external temperature. The hypothalamus supervises this through a 'temperature eye', a group of nerve cells which can measure very exactly the temperature of the blood. This works like a thermostat. If the body temperature diverges too far from the desired level, the temperature eye switches on the heating or the cooling. The body is heated by priming the metabolism, but must be cooled if we start to sweat. Warmth is required for the water secreted to evaporate, and this is withdrawn from the overheated body.

The hypothalamus supervises input and output in a similar way. Special groups of nerve cells make us feel hungry or full up, while others produce thirst or increase the kidney's action after an excessive intake of fluid. We feel hunger in the stomach and thirst in the mouth, but both stomach and mouth sound the alarm on instructions from the hypothalamus, which signals to them when it is time to rumble with hunger or feel dry with thirst.

Considering the large numbers of overweight people these days, it might seem that the hypothalamus is not much good as regulator of food intake. Probably, however, it is merely designed for a different way of life from ours today. At least in the affluent society of the West the abundance of appetite-producing stimuli seems to overtax it. With animals at large, which are thus not surrounded by constant delicacies, the hypothalamus functions perfectly.

But a slight current from correctly placed electrodes drastically disturbs animals' normal feeding behaviour. When an eating system in the hypothalamus is stimulated, a well-fed animal which has had a good meal will indulge in unrestained over-eating. Stimulation of a satiation system makes a hungry animal spit out food it already has in its mouth.

Many of the discoveries about the hypothalamus, and also about neighbouring areas in the brain's interior, were made through experiments in electrical stimulation at specific points; at others it produced vomiting, defecation or urination; at others again, feelings of pleasure, rage or fear.

Control of breathing, heart action and blood pressure, digestion and vomiting, have already been mentioned as functions of the brain stem, and it may seem confusing that the hypothalamus is also concerned with them; but the brain's structures are not at all like a chemist's shelves with one kind of pillbox neatly arranged next to another. Different parts of the brain sometimes work together in a fairly inscrutable partnership. There is thus no contradiction to the finding that operations on different parts of the brain influence one and the same bodily function or produce the same behaviour.

To carry out its wide-ranging functions the hypothalamus has at its disposal besides the nerve network the body's second communication system, the hormones. They are the couriers in a system which regulates the activity of the various organs in the body and adjusts them to each other. While the nervous system makes possible quick reactions, such as we need, say, when we suddenly have to step on the brakes, the hormonal system controls mainly operations where steadiness is more important than speed, which ensure the regular course of highly complex chemical processes.

The hypothalamus is in the most favourable place to exert its influence on the hormonal system. Directly adjacent, connected with it by a short pathway, is the pituitary gland which, despite its small size (about that of a pea), occupies a unique position among the hormonal glands. The hormones it secretes into the blood-stream control most of the other hormonal glands, such as the thyroid, the adrenal cortex, the gonads; the pituitary itself is controlled by the hypothalamus. Two hormones which are released by the pituitary even come direct from the hypothalamus. One, vasopressin, increases the blood pressure and ensures that the body does not secrete more water than is necessary. The other, oxytocin, plays a rôle at birth, causing the mother to contract and thus bringing on the labour.

The thalamus

The thalamus consists of two egg-shaped masses of grey

brain substance about an inch and a half long. It is often described as a great switchboard—but it is an extremely complicated sort of switchboard.

The various areas of the cerebral cortex exchange information with each other partly by way of the thalamus. They do not have direct contact even when right by each other (like the motor and the sensory thalamus) and designed for continual close contact. The thalamus is a station for the collection and distribution of information, and so that it should all duly arrive, some of the different areas of the cerebral cortex are represented by particular parts of the thalamus—here there are 'shelves at the chemist's' to a limited degree.

The idea everyone has of his own body, an indispensable condition for all movements, seems to be lodged in the thalamus. Electrical stimulations of the appropriate areas which have to be carried out for diagnostic reasons lead to the patient's feeling a strange alienation from individual parts of his body. Face or tongue or limbs may seem suddenly distorted for several minutes. If the appropriate regions of the thalamus have to be destroyed to relieve patients of illnesses, parts of the body may for days or weeks feel deformed, bigger, smaller or heavier than usual.

The importance of the thalamus is not confined to being a message centre for the cerebrum. Signals come into it from all areas of the brain and the body, and these stimulations have an interacting influence, so it is also an integration and co-ordination centre. There is clear evidence that external stimuli received by the body, perceptions of touch, pain and temperature, and also signals coming from the body itself, visceral sensations, perceptions of taste and balance, are effectively 'coloured' in the thalamus, ie. they are connected with pleasure, aversion and other feelings.

It is still very hard to form even a moderately satisfactory idea of the function of the thalamus, as of the other parts of the brain described in this chapter. An impression of the uncertainty felt even by experts is given in the testimony of the Russian scientist Vladimir Smirnov, who has made a special study of the thalamus:

'Modern conceptions of the physiological bases of man's psychic activity can be successfully developed only if there is a great mass of facts on the part played by the thalamus in the system mechanisms of the psychic functions. This material is for the moment insufficient . . . New data . . . are evidence of its highly complicated and differentiated rôle in the regulation of the inner centres, which are of great importance for the control of the waking condition and the emotions; they are evidence, too, of its undoubted rôle in the activity of the brain systems which give sensations an emotional tone and place them in a context of the external and internal (bodily) space.'

The importance of the thalamus cannot be fully appreciated without taking into account a great many observations made on human patients as well as on animals. Smirnov noted that during stimulation in the front part of the thalamus patients suffered from loss of memory. W. R. Hess, the pioneer of electrical stimulation in the lower regions of the brain, put cats to sleep by stimuli in the thalamus. Brain surgeons in various countries have proved that deliberate removal of certain regions of the thalamus could help patients with severe illnesses. For instance, it stopped excessive movements of particular parts of the body which the patients could not control, and so got rid of extremely severe pain.

Rolf Hassler, of the Max Planck Institute for Brain Research in Frankfurt, observed that patients whose thalamus was exposed to slight electrical stimuli uttered sounds, words or even short sentences, like 'Stop!', 'Keep moving' or 'Go into the cellar and fetch potatoes'. Other stimulation points in the thalamus produced movements, even when the patients had been expressly forbidden to move.

A specially astonishing reaction was obtained by stimulating the region in the thalamus where nerve cells project to the area of the cerebral cortex responsible for controlling neck and head movements: over a quarter of the patients stimulated there burst out laughing. It was no empty laughter; they reported feeling amused despite their far from comfortable situation on the operating table. Asked what had made them laugh, they gave reasons like: 'Directly the stimulus starts, I find everything so funny' or 'I simply can't help laughing, I have a feeling of amusement, but don't know what's causing it.' Right by the laughter region the current produced mainly smiles. Brain researchers have been able to cause muscle movements by electrical stimuli at the cerebral cortex, but never laughter or smiles. It evidently needed particular influences in the thalamus to co-ordinate muscle movements which animated laughter and at the same time connect them with the appropriate mood.

The limbic system

Deep in the interior of the cerebrum, bordering brain stem and diencephalon, there are important nerve centres which play a quite different rôle from the cortex. Their function is rather similar to the functions of the hypothalamus and brain stem; they seem to have less communication than the thalamus with the cerebral cortex. They are called the 'limbic system' (from the Latin word *limbus*=border); and here too electrical stimuli or injuries can produce disorders of breathing, circulation, digestion and similar functions. The stimulation points for the various functions are distributed over the whole limbic system and often overlap. Important elements in our affective and sexual behaviour are regulated in the limbic system, and our memory is decisively stamped here.

Electrical stimulation of structures in the limbic system can produce dangerous increases in aggressive behaviour with animals and men, and also abnormal tameness or lack of drive. Similar effects occur from injuries men have suffered in the limbic system through tumours or haemorrhages. In severe cases it may lead to violent outbursts of rage for no cause. Such patients, driven to frenzy by their brain damage, will yell loudly and attack any of the people round them, biting them and trying to throttle them. These fits, reaching real mania in advanced stages, occur through a brain inflammation in the limbic system. Other changes, too, in mood and emotion have been observed by brain researchers after electrical stimulation or disease processes in the limbic system: fear and terror, sadness and aversion—indeed they are almost always unpleasant in character.

With laboratory animals and also patients, disorders in the limbic system can lead to an enormous increase in sexual drive. Under an irresistible compulsion such patients will indiscriminately seek sexual contacts or indulge extravagantly in masturbation. Yet they do not experience any of the pleasure normally so much prized, but find their compulsion extremely tormenting. Sometimes a deviation in direction is involved, so that they feel compelled to homosexual, sadistic or exhibitionist actions. Apart from the increase in sexual drive, the limbic system, like the brain stem and diencephalon, does also contain pleasure centres, which animals and men like having stimulated.

There is a part of the limbic system which imaginative anatomists decided to call 'hippocampus' (sea-horse). Brain researchers were surprised to find that, in an area concerned with automatically controlled bodily functions and with emotions, the hippocampus had great importance for the memory. In the 'fifties, hoping to help acute epileptic and psychotic patients, surgeons removed parts of the cerebrum which also included the hippocampus in each hemisphere. Without a hippocampus, it turned out, the patients were no longer capable of enlarging their memory with new impressions. They reacted intelligently and behaved normally, but their memory was confined to the immediate present. They kept on having to be introduced to people they had only just met; every day they would read the same magazine with lively interest. Before a test they could safely be told all the answers; after a short time they would not have any recollection of them.

It has not yet been discovered exactly what part the hippocampus plays in memory. Many brain researchers suppose there is a sort of attention mechanism there, its function being to select the impressions continually flowing in to the brain as memories to be imprinted in the whole 'memory'. Others think the brain without a hippocampus is capable of enlarging the memory with new impressions, but that the hippocampus is needed to recall the information from the memory to consciousness. In any case, without a hippocampus man lacks something essential.

Man, horse and crocodile

From forms of life with simply structured brains, man has developed through a long succession of animal ancestors. When he set about seizing power on earth, nature did not at first make him a completely new brain, but equipped him with a further development of the ancestors' simple structures. Many parts which have survived from those still do service, though with some changes, in the human brain. To quote Paul MacLean of the National Institutes of Health in Bethesda, Maryland:

'Man finds himself in the situation that Nature has equipped him in essentials with three different brains, which—despite the difference in their structure—have to function and communicate together. The oldest is like a reptile's, the second derives from lower mammals, and the last is a late mammal development which has really made man into man. In allegorical terms: when the psychotherapist asks the patient to lie down on the couch, we must imagine that he is inviting him to lie down by a horse and by a crocodile.'

Of course man's ancestors do not directly include crocodiles and horses, but they do include fishes, reptiles, shrewlike insect-eaters and monkeys. It is obvious which are the old parts in our brain: above all, brain stem, hypothalamus and limbic system (the thalamus evolved later). The regulation mechanisms for the smooth running of bodily functions and the control systems for emotions are older than the systems for thinking. The thinking apparatus has taken between half a million and two million years to develop to an effective instrument—a sudden explosion considering the time-spans otherwise needed by nature for important evolutionary processes.

Harmonious results are scarcely to be expected from an explosion, so we should not be surprised that the older parts of our brain are not yet rightly adapted to the new ones. They seem, Arthur Koestler has said, to lead 'a kind of agonised co-existence—when not in acute conflict with each other'.

Certainly there are very frequent conflicts in man's brain. The parts we have inherited from the anthropoid apes react with emotions as they always did, where it would be better for them to leave it to the thinking regions of the cerebrum to find solutions for difficulties. Often enough the new, human brain does not get its way, as everyone knows: emotions easily overcome wisdom.

The dangerous thing is that when the old parts win the victory, they use the thinking capacity of the new parts, in order to assert the power of the emotions, not to seek the path of wisdom. We see examples of this every day in muggings and riots, revolutions and dictatorships, wars and genocide. The worst cases get into the history books.

Since hydrogen bombs were developed, man has been threatened with total self-destruction. The swamping of understanding by aggressiveness, in view of the technical possibilities achieved, has become an intolerable threat to humanity.

9

Electrical Manipulation

George Orwell's 'Big Brother' in 1984 keeps his subjects under constant watch by television cameras. In 1949, the year when Orwell wrote his grim vision of the future, W. R. Hess was awarded the Nobel Prize for medicine for his pioneering experiments in brain stimulation, which had already been going for some time but had not received much public notice. His work revealed the possibilities of such stimulation; and the ideas developed since then make Orwell's fantasies look quite old-fashioned.

Already in the 'fifties the American electronic engineer Curtiss R. Schafer found it 'economically quite worth considering' to plant hundreds of electrodes into the brains of children directly after birth and thereafter direct the children by radio signals. Such radio-controlled children would be far cheaper to produce and maintain than robots: 'to construct a simple mechanical machine man on present standards costs about ten times as much as the birth and breeding of a child up to his sixteenth year.' And in 1968 the magazine *Newsweek* commented: 'In 1984 it seems Big Brother will no longer have to watch. He'll just tune in and turn people on or off.'

We are coming closer to 1984 without the menacing aspects of brain stimulation looking in too great danger of being realised. All the same José Delgado reported in 1970 having given a computer at Yale the task of taming a self-assertive and aggressive young chimpanzee called Paddy with the aid of brain stimulations, and making him quiet and obedient. After a few days the computer had fulfilled its assignment, and it took about a fortnight after it was switched off before Paddy had recovered his spirit.

The principle was simple. Delgado installed on Paddy's head a transmitter and receiver the size of a cigarette lighter, which he called a 'stimoceiver'. This was connected with electrodes leading deep into Paddy's brain, and he was in radio contact with the computer. He fed it with the pattern of electric currents from Paddy's brain, and in return received signals which he transmitted into the brain. The computer received a special input from an area of the limbic system which the anatomists have christened the *amygdala* (from the Latin for walnut) because of its shape. These currents showed a typical pattern when Paddy behaved aggressively. The computer, programmed accordingly, analysed the currents, and directly it discovered signs of aggressiveness, sent signals to the stimoceiver which transmitted the signals into a particular area of the brain stem. This brain stimulation produced an unpleasant feeling, and Paddy's brain soon grasped the connection between that feeling and his aggressive behaviour: he became mild as a lamb.

A model for future efforts to turn young thugs into peaceful members of society? Why not, if it can help both the victims by stopping the violence and the thugs who are now outlawed because of it? But where do you draw the line? Brain-stimuli suppressing aggressiveness for sons who oppose their fathers? Definitely not. For rebellious students more concerned with 'demos' than with their studies? For political extremists with respectable motives whose ideological fanaticism may have even more brutal effects than are caused by the thugs? For psychopaths—clockwork oranges galore? Who is to decide?

Plans to make the agents and advocates of violence pacific, on the model of Paddy or by other operations, are likely to produce more aggressiveness (between supporters and opponents of the idea) than will be removed by the treatment of those who need it or are deemed to need it. Early thought is essential on how such unwanted effects might be eliminated.

Electrodes to fight aggression

Many other impressive demonstrations have been given, besides Paddy's taming, of aggressive animals suddenly becoming peaceful through deliberate brain stimuli. Unmanageable monkeys, who usually could not be fed without safety precautions being taken, directly the current flowed into the brain would even allow the food to be taken out of their mouths. At the University of California in Los Angeles Carmine D. Clemente got cats to let go of rats they were just about to kill. A burst of current into the right centre made the cats completely forget their intention. Without taking any further notice of their victims, they crept away and lay down to sleep in a corner of the cage.

José Delgado, a Spaniard by birth, a neuropsychologist with great physical courage and a flair for causing sensations, went into the bull-ring at Cordoba armed only with a minitransmitter, and let the bull charge him. He had previously planted an electrode in its brain, and when the bull was only two yards away, he pressed the transmitting knob. It immediately stopped in its tracks.

In another experiment he planted an electrode in the brain of a monkey called Ali, the tyrannical head of a family of four. Ali's mate Elsa, the most subordinate member of the family, quickly learnt to mollify the tyrant by working an electric switch near the manger. In the end she reached the point of deliberately defying him and only checking him in his fury at the last second with the aid of the switch.

Such a pacifier switch would no doubt seem desirable to many who suffer under an insupportable boss or a dictatorial parent. Obviously the method with which Elsa protected herself from Ali offers no practical solution for human relations; but doctors have begun to use electrical brain stimulation at least on patients with extreme inclinations to violence.

Over two hundred men and women who were continually making unnecessary attacks on other people were investigated and treated at Massachussetts General Hospital in Boston, where Frank R. Erwin is director of a centre for psychiatric research. In a number of cases electrical stimulation of the brain was a considerable help in discovering the cause of the unwarranted violence and cutting it out.

One of the patients was a young woman who without any reason had already made twelve attacks on others, including a woman who accidentally touched her arm in the cloak-room of a restaurant and whom she almost killed. By brain stimulation with electrodes Ervin found out which place in the brain was responsible for this unrestrained aggressiveness. When the electrode was in the right place, she promptly became worked up as soon as the current was switched on. The excitement ended abruptly when a point was stimulated adjacent to the centre which produced the aggressiveness. Once recognised, the dangerous brain tissue, a tiny region, could be destroyed, and the tendency to violence disappeared.

There was also a very talented engineer who had fits of rage in which he sometimes hurled his wife across the room. Ervin planted in his head an electrode through which a small place deep in the brain could regularly be stimulated —with the result that the fits stopped. An operation seemed indicated for a permanent solution, and this had the success desired: it was some years ago, and since then no outbursts of uncontrollable rage have occurred. A similar operation stopped a mother in Boston from periodically beating her twelve-year-old son almost unconscious in her frantic rage. Dangerous aggression has also been damped down in other cases. Ten seconds of brain stimuli at the right place, Delgado reported on one patient, suppressed aggressive behaviour for up to forty-eight hours.

What chance for dictators?

Knowledge about pleasure centres has also been used clinically. Robert Heath in New Orleans and other researchers after him have planted into many people's heads brain electrodes leading to these centres. The patients have included schizophrenics resistant to all attempts at treatment, sufferers from persistent depressions and compulsion neuroses, but also cancer patients with unrelievable pain. Directly the current is switched on, they feel the beneficial effect: despair and hopelessness disappear, intolerable pain dissolves or at least is alleviated. The feeling of well-being varies according to which pleasure centre is touched. In extreme cases the brain stimulus, as one depressive patient said, is 'better than sex'.

A dictator who was put in the position of rewarding 'good behaviour' by granting pleasure feelings could easily achieve whatever he wanted. An idea of the possibilities is given by an experiment carried out in America with a monkey, which had an electrode in its brain leading to a pleasure centre. The current for stimulating the centre was provided by a photo-cell buckled on to the monkey. Thus equipped, he was sent off to a destination unknown to him. He arrived there safely.

The photo-cell was in fact attached to his body in such a way that the sun shone on it while the direction was right. If the monkey strayed from his course, no more sunlight came on to the photo-cell, no more current flowed into the electrode, and the pleasure centre remained unstimulated. The monkey, 'hooked' on pleasure feelings, reverted as quickly as possible to the right direction.

Understandably, no medical application has yet been found for the possibility of stimulating aversion centres in the brain and so producing discomfort, pain or fear— although this could of course be used as a form of aversion therapy to make alcoholics, for instance, dislike drinking. In any case such feelings can undoubtedly be produced by stimulation of these centres. Experiments on monkeys subjected to it have shown how extremely effective the stimuli are for punishment purposes. The monkeys could pull a lever to switch on the stimulus themselves, and soon afterwards the current began to flow. They were then constantly occupied with fruitless attempts to get rid of the tormenting discomfort. After three hours they were completely distracted and irritable. They refused to eat or to co-operate any further. Several died. But when a pleasure centre was stimulated afterwards, the monkeys which had been made ill regained their health and spirits within a few minutes.

Like most animals, man lives in groups. Anyone who wanted to manipulate people by brain stimuli could start at this point too. For, as researchers have repeatedly found in experiments with animals, influencing a single member of the group by brain electrodes can drastically alter the behaviour of others in the group—especially when brain stimulation produces aggressiveness.

Delgado put a cat and a kitten together on a platform. They got on well until a brain stimulus made the kitten aggressive. Directly the current was switched on, it began to spit, showed its claws, and attacked the cat, which responded, after a moment of surprise, by defending itself. The fight broke off at once when the brain stimulus was stopped, and restarted when the current flowed again. After the kitten, under the compulsion of some current, had several times repeated its sudden attack, the good relations between the two cats were shattered. From then on they watched each other with hostility.

R. Apfelbach at the University of California in Berkeley upset the social life of a gibbon family by using a succession of electrical stimuli at short intervals to make one of the gibbons howl loudly and behave aggressively. 'If structures which generate aggressive behaviour and noise-making are stimulated,' he reported, 'normal group behaviour disintegrates.'

Electrical stimuli can dethrone leaders and bring to power previously obedient followers. In Yerkes Regional Primate Research Centre, Bryan W. Robinson stimulated the sexuality of a lower-ranking chimpanzee in such a way that the former underling asserted himself against the chimpanzee lord and forced him into the rôle of a spectator. It is hard to say whether this procedure could be adapted in human society for humiliating paladins fallen from grace or rivals beaten in the fight for power; no doubt there are simpler methods already available for carrying out such purposes.

But suppressing aggressiveness, producing feelings of pleasure or of fear and pain, destroying the normal fabric of unpopular groups—such attacks on the human psyche, technically quite possible today by brain stimulation, might be very attractive to a dictator. Two of the possibilities of manipulating minds could even be praised as philanthropic ideas; who would deny that it is a worthy aim to give people more peace and well-being?

The experts are divided on the expediency and necessity, advantages and disadvantages, of electrical brain manipulation in human society. Many, like Nobel prize-winner Sir John Eccles, fear it more than the atom bomb; others are concerned that efforts to civilise the human psyche might come too late. The former see a wide extension of brain stimuli as the end of human life, the latter as the beginning.

Delgado, called by the British scientific journalist Nigel

Calder 'the prophet in chief of a better world through brain electrodes', thinks there are great prospects from mind manipulation. He looks forward to a human society 'psycho-civilised' for the very first time through brain stimulation and other influencing techniques. Considering human aggressiveness, Arthur Koestler has said, such a development cannot start soon enough.

Most researchers, however, do not believe it will be possible to carry out on a large scale such controversial incursions into the human brain. Pessimistic predictions that whole populations might be enslaved through 'soul manipulation' are rejected as futile by Seymour Kety of Massachusetts General Hospital on the grounds that 'anyone influential enough to get an entire population to consent to having electrodes put into their heads would already have achieved his goal without firing a single volt'. But this reflection starts from the premise that a dictator would suddenly try to introduce soul manipulation with a people unprepared and unmotivated for the innovation.

Kety does not take into account that it would probably creep in, starting in hospitals, and then perhaps going on to prisons, where brain stimulation might also be shown to be desirable. Brain electrodes, positioned in pleasure centres by specialised pseudo-doctors, might in fringe zones of society compete as fashionable joy-bringers with hashish, LSD and heroin. Once established, brain stimulation might gradually become acceptable, to a degree which would eventually allow the dictator to take the plunge into total manipulation.

This also, of course, is mere speculation. We know today the uses to which electrical brain stimulation can be put. No one knows what the future may hold; only vigilance can protect us from unpleasant surprises.

IO

Chemical Manipulation

Scientists found they could exert a profound influence on laboratory animals not only by electric current but also by chemical substances introduced into the brain with precise aim and the right dose. This chemical brain stimulation brought new and surprising results; and even though they were obtained exclusively on animals, there is no doubt that basically they are valid also for men. It is true that the manipulation possibilities which cause anxiety to expert 'futurologists' do not yet include 'brain-drops' to make men controllable in a similar way. But an application of the discoveries, say in overcoming aggression, seems by no means out of the question.

When in the 'fifties the first researchers started on chemical stimulation experiments, they were wanting to obtain even more information than electric stimulations could give, about the structures hidden deep in the brain's interior. All the nerve cells near the tip of an electrode react to electric current. They hoped for more finely differentiated reactions from chemical stimuli depending on the kind of chemicals used. These hopes were fulfilled, but not immediately.

A successful chemical brain stimulation was reported in

1953 by the Swede Bengt Andersson. In his experiments he injected a five per cent salt solution into a particular area of goats' brains, in the middle of the hypothalamus. The effect was seen at once: the goats drank a lot of water.

Systematic investigations were started a year later by the American psychologist Alan E. Fisher. First at McGill University, Montreal, later at the University of Wisconsin, and above all at the University of Pittsburgh, he placed fine tubes of stainless steel in the brains of hundreds of rats, and through these tubes he could make chemical substances act exactly at the point desired.

In a first series of experiments with male rats, Fisher poured the male sex hormone, testosterone, into various places in the hypothalamus and adjoining parts of the brain. He naturally expected that, provided they were stimulated in the right area, they would show an unusually strong sexual drive. But when after several failures a rat reacted to the hormone, something unexpected happened. Seconds after the hormone injection began, the rat began to run excitedly round the cage. Assuming the testosterone was already working, as he had envisaged, Fisher put into the cage a female unresponsive at the time to male advances. The male, Fisher hoped, would prove its increased sexuality by ignoring the female's unwilling attitude. Male rats are not normally so inconsiderate.

But this male had something other than sex in mind. He caught her by the tail with his teeth and dragged her across the cage into a corner. She ran away as soon as she could. This performance was repeated several times. Finally he took hold of her by the neck, as mother rats are accustomed to carry their young, and put her in the corner. 'I was extremely startled,' Fisher recalled later, 'and so no doubt was the female rat.'

When he had recovered from his astonishment, it occurred to him how similar the behaviour shown by the male under the influence of testosterone was to maternal behaviour. He took the female out of the cage and instead put shavings in and new-born rat babies. The male rat promptly built a nest out of the shavings, into which he carried the young. The strange effect of the male sex hormone disappeared about half an hour after the injection. But a new dose of it, administered in the same way, turned the rat back immediately into a solicitous mother.

Further experiments confirmed the first observation. At the same stimulation point, directly in front of the hypothalamus, tiny quantities of testosterone produced maternal behaviour in both male and female rats. Fisher's original assumption, that the male sex hormone would lead to striking male sexual behaviour, was in the end proved correct. At a point very near the first it had the effect he had once expected. No matter whether the other rat in the cage was male or female, the rat under the hormonal brain stimulus tried to mount his partner. But another strange result occurred: female rats, when the hormone took effect on the same stimulation point, were impelled to the same behaviour. 'One heroic female,' Fisher reported, 'in tests carried out every other day, stuck to this male behaviour for eight weeks.'

When, however, the hormone was injected into a place between the two stimulation points (for maternal and for male sexual behaviour), some rats demonstrated a curious behaviour mixture: they looked after the babies and were at the same time bent on copulating with any accessible partner. A male would repeatedly try to mount unresponsive females or other males, while holding a young rat with his teeth.

Such results suggest that the male and female brain, at least in rats, must be very similarly organised in the parts responsible for sex-specific behaviour; although it is hard to understand why male hormone should also produce female (maternal) behaviour. For an explanation Fisher could only point to the fact that testosterone and the female sex hormone progesterone are chemically closely related.

In the same sort of way as he had influenced sexual behaviour with a sex hormone, he hoped also to manipulate chemically the feeding habits of his rats. With two hormones of the pancreas, insulin, which reduces the blood sugar, and its opposite, glucagon, he intended to act on the feeding and satiation centres in the hypothalamus. It sounded a plausible idea. But however precisely he applied the hormones, it did not show the slightest effect.

A Yale student, Sebastian P. Grossman, discovered the trick whereby hunger and thirst could be chemically produced. He worked with two substances which are regularly to be found in the brain, noradrenalin and acetylcholine. He poured some of the former into a region of the brain right above the hypothalamus, and satiated rats started to eat again. He injected the latter into exactly the same place, and they began to drink; in fact they developed a colossal thirst. Whereas rats normally take in 25–35 c.c. a day, these drank double that amount in an hour under the influence of the acetylcholine.

This showed that different chemical substances at the same place in the brain can produce different effects. It also showed that in the rat brain, especially in the limbic system, there are many points at which noradrenalin and acetylcholine can become effective. Fisher and his colleague John N. Coury now made an extensive search through brain injections for hunger and thirst points. They put together the points discovered in three-dimensional maps. During these investigations Fisher found a place at which he could even produce three different effects: acetylcholine made the rat drink, noradrenalin made it eat, and testosterone made it build a nest.

When Fisher and Coury brought other animals into their investigations, there was again a different result from what they had expected. Following their discoveries on rats, they tried to make up a thirst map in the cat brain as well. But however often they injected acetylcholine into the brains of cats, the cats never became thirsty. Instead the injections made them angry or fearful, they became sleepy or fell into a trance.

In a certain region of the cats' temporal lobe, acetyl-choline produced lasting changes in their behaviour. Originally friendly cats became vicious and attacked the rats and dogs as well as men and other cats. They also suffered from epileptic fits. The effects of a single injection of acetylcholine at this point were still showing after months.

With serotonin, a third substance to be found in the brain, the temperature regulation in cats' hypothalamus could be influenced. Injected into the front part of the hypothalamus, it made the body temperature rise and brought the cats out in shivers.

Killers and pacifists

Interesting as these and other observations are, the chemical stimulation of the brain has so far raised more questions than it has answered. We are still missing a key discovery to reveal the principle behind the findings, which at present appear rather unconnected. Only one important result from more recent research should be mentioned: it has been possible by chemical brain manipulation to make 'bloodthirsty' rats peaceful and also to arouse in 'tolerant' rats the urge to kill.

The American psychologists Douglas Smith, Melvyn King and Bartley Hoebel at Princeton University sorted rats by their behaviour towards mice into 'killers' and 'pacifists'. Most rats do not kill mice without reason, but many do, if they can catch them, through a bite in the neck. To test the rats, the psychologists assigned a mouse to each rat. Rats put in the killer category were those which killed the mouse within less than two minutes on three successive days. A rat was acknowledged as a pacifist if it never killed a mouse after seventeen opportunities.

Such a peaceful disposition was abruptly transformed into murderousness when the researchers injected a synthetic substance called carbachol, with an effect similar to that of acetylcholine, at a place in the hypothalamus. The rats treated in this way finished off the wretched mice as quickly, motivelessly and in the same manner as the born killers did. But it needed the right substance in the right place. Salt solution and various other substances injected in the same place did not change the rats' behaviour. When the carbachol was injected more than a fraction of an inch from the effective point, the pacifist rats remained as peaceful as ever.

The reverse effect, taking blood-lust away from the killers, was achieved by Smith and his colleagues through injecting into the hypothalamus the substance methylatropine; this removes the effect of acetylcholine which the killer rats may have in excessive quantity in the 'killing centre'. At any rate the researchers observed a prompt effect of the methylatropine: the previously murderous rats now approached the mice peacefully, sniffed at them in a friendly way, and did nothing to hurt them. The aggression-inhibiting action of an injection of methylatropine lasted between six and sixteen minutes. Then the killer rats revealed their vicious side again. Filled with blood-lust by carbachol, pacifists took three-quarters of an hour on average to revert to their peaceful selves.

The researchers concluded from their findings that acetylcholine plays an important part in an innate system for killing and that there may be a similar system with other species as well. In view of the tantalising differences shown particularly with chemical brain stimulation between different species, this conclusion can only be regarded as a working hypothesis well worth trying out.

The same reservation should be made about the comment by Smith, King and Hoebel that these thoughts point to 'the practical possibility that pharmacological manipulation of such a system might be used for the treatment of morbidly aggressive behaviour'. In other words, anti-aggression drugs seem conceivable.

Alas, should we pursue our speculations into the future, past some 'ifs' and 'buts', the opposite of a pacifist-making drug seems conceivable too: an inciting drug which turns sensible citizens into ruthless killers. Demagogy in bottles, perfect, irresistible and non-addictive—this too could result from investigations on the chemistry of the brain.

Again and again we see the two faces of brain research. Humanity will have to rally all the vigilance and wisdom of which it is capable, if it wishes to benefit by the promising discoveries and avoid the menacing consequences.

I I

Psychoactive Drugs

'The drink has swept me away like a hurricane . . . One half of my being leaves the two worlds behind . . . I have surpassed in greatness this heaven and this earth . . . I realise I have drunk Soma.'

This is from one of the hundred and twenty Indian hymns, over three thousand years old, in which the authors of the *Rig-Veda*, most ancient of Hindu holy books, celebrate the magic drink Soma, which makes people feel they are literally growing 'above themselves' and are like gods.

Man has a primeval longing for a better and more beautiful life than the real world can offer him. Everywhere and in all ages human beings must have been attracted by the idea that at least for a while they could escape from the cares and sorrows of everyday life. In all civilisations means were found by which people, even if they could not change their natures, could for a short time so transform themselves that they basked in an ecstasy of bliss.

The art of making alcoholic drinks was probably discovered in prehistoric times. Four thousand years ago the Sumerians brewed beer in Babylon. Hemp, the source of hashish and marihuana, was listed over five thousand years

ago, in the herbal manual of a Chinese emperor. It is hard
to say how long drugs have been prized in the New World,
but Columbus reported that the inhabitants of the part of
the continent he discovered smoked tobacco leaves. When
the Spanish conquistadors conquered Peru and Mexico at
the beginning of the sixteenth century, the natives of the
Inca empire ate cocoa leaves, the Aztecs ate an intoxicating
cactus decoction or 'holy mushrooms'.

Everywhere and in all ages, as far back as our sources
reach, man has tried to interfere in the normal course of his
psychological functions, in fact to manipulate his brain.
Psychoactive drugs were once considered divine gifts which
one used gratefully, or as the temptations of evil spirits to
which one succumbed. Today we know that they are
substances which, through the structure of their molecules,
influence chemical processes in the brain.

Massive brain manipulation was taking place, then, long
before the chemical manipulators had any idea what the
brain meant for them. The remarkable experiences induced
by drugs, one might with hindsight have expected, would
have made it easier for leading thinkers of past ages to achieve
realistic conceptions of the human mind. But instead the
idea was proclaimed, and constantly reiterated, that mind,
let alone soul, was fundamentally different both from the
body it inhabited and from the rest of the world, that it
obeyed completely different laws from those governing
matter. Although the experience was easily accessible to
anyone, it was scarcely registered that a small quantity of
suitable matter, like a drug, could have a dramatic influence
on mind and psyche (personality).

Basically, little has changed for most people even today.
They are still completely 'thrown' by the idea that the only
reason why tobacco and coffee, whisky and wine, hashish
and heroin, can have the effect they do is that the human
mind is thoroughly involved in the physical universe and is
at least to a considerable extent the result of normal chemical

and physical processes in the brain.

Yet at no previous time have there been so many substances which influence the brain's functions. The old 'drugs', tobacco, coffee and tea, alcoholic drinks for every taste, are within almost everyone's reach; anyone who wants hashish (pot) or LSD knows how to get hold of them; so far the authorities have striven in vain to dam the black market channels through which the specially dangerous heroin flows in. There are many other psychoactive substances which are used, and often misused, as medicines: sleeping tablets and tablets to keep you awake, tranquillisers and anti-depressants, pain killers and pills to suppress excessive appetite. Drugs which can untie psychological knots or make possible effective treatment of patients with schizophrenia, manias and acute depressions are among the most important new developments of medicine in the last two decades.

All these substances are among the psychoactive drugs. In the wider sense that term includes alcohol and nicotine, hashish and heroin, even though they have not advanced medicine at all, and in fact raise serious health problems. But they are as interesting to brain researchers as drugs which can heal sick minds. Even the latter can produce as well as remove disorders in psychic functioning: there is no sharp line to be drawn here, or between 'useful' and 'harmful' psychoactive drugs. How the effect is to be assessed depends on many other factors, above all on the dose, but also on the subject's personality, physical constitution, condition at the time, and the general situation. If a bottle of beer in the evening removes difficulties in going to sleep, that may be a healing and desirable effect of alcohol. With morphine it is generally possible to alleviate even the most intolerable pain, an extremely positive effect, especially for patients with not long to live. But its use has to be controlled very strictly indeed because of its great addictiveness. The use and abuse of psychoactive drugs, in fact, is notoriously one of the thorniest of today's social problems.

Drugs of former times

The ingenuity man has shown from ancient times in discovering ways of influencing the brain's activity is astonishing. With sure detective powers inhabitants of countries all over the world tracked down the products of nature which were available for brain manipulation. The observation that a liquid containing carbohydrate, certainly designed for nourishment, could be turned by fermentation into an intoxicating (alcoholic) drink, may have come fairly easily and been made independently in many different places. But from the vast number of plants which cover the earth the natives also discovered the particular ones which had interesting effects on the brain. Moreover they recognised by the active content which parts of these drugs produced the pleasantest effects, and how best to prepare and enjoy them.

Opium, for instance, is obtained from the capsules of a kind of poppy; you scrape them just before they are ripe, and next morning scrape off the milky juice which has come out and has meanwhile dried up. Hashish comes from hemp plants, and only from female ones which grow in warm climates. When they are in bloom, glandular hairs develop at their shoots; it is the resin coming out of the hairs which contains the drug.

People looking for interesting brain stimuli discovered caffein in a whole number of plants: not only in the seeds of the coffee tree but also in leaf-buds and leaves of the tea plant, in leaves and branches of the mast tree, in the seeds of the cola tree and of the guarana liana. These species of plants are not connected, and they are found in regions of the earth very far away from each other. The coffee tree comes from Abyssinia, the tea plant from South-east Asia, mast tree and guarana liana grow in South America, cola tree in West Africa.

The Incas or their predecessors had found out that eating

the leaves of the coconut tree, which is very prolific in the Andes, could produce a euphoric mood. Their successors made things easier for themselves by chewing dried coconut leaves with some chalk and vegetable ashes. Indians in the south of North America discovered that a small thornless cactus called peyote and a number of nondescript-looking fungi caused striking hallucinations.

Inhabitants of all five continents found that many plants of the deadly nightshade family (which includes potatoes, tomatoes and tobacco) contained hallucinogens. In Europe the nightshade varieties of belladonna, henbane and thorn-apple provided the active ingredients of the 'magic ointment' with which at the end of the Middle Ages women especially obtained erotic visions: in the spirit of the time these were seen as a form of intercourse with the devil, and they quite often led to the stake.

In Europe today there are no longer any enthusiasts for nightshade drugs or for the fungus fly agaric, which rots unwanted in our woods because it is considered so poisonous. Many tribes in Siberia, however, valued so highly the hallucinations which can be produced by fly agaric, eaten in moderation, that the fungi are rarities today and can be traded against reindeer and reindeer skins. Necessity is the mother of invention: the Siberian peoples discovered that a large part of the active substance was discharged unaltered with the urine, so that a dearly bought fungus ration could be used for several 'trips'. According to a well-based theory of Gordon Watson, the American researcher into drug fungi, Soma, to which the ancient Hindus devoted so many hymns, was a preparation of fly agaric.

Morphine, heroin, cocaine

The chemists' art has very much extended the possibilities for manipulation. The psychoactive natural products are complemented today by an abundance of other psychoactive drugs. Some of these are isolated as effective agents from the natural products and so represent a concentration of drug-forming substances, but the majority are synthesised and without a prototype in nature. The chemists' retorts have given birth to products very important for medicine and also to substances which can be dangerously misused.

In 1808 Friedrich Sertürner, a young chemist's assistant in the Westphalian town of Paderborn, succeeded in isolating the most important active substance of opium. He called the white powder he had found 'morphium' after Morpheus, Greek god of sleep. Its technical chemical name today is morphine.

This solved an important medical problem. Opium, already valued as a powerful pain-killer by ancient civilisations, may contain varying amounts of this active substance and of other substances also acting on the organism; so it was always inclined to kill the patient as well as the pain. But now a new problem arose: the danger of addiction, which had long been recognised, was even greater with morphine than with opium.

Since then chemists have made continual efforts to find drugs as effective or even more so in the fight against pain, without the patients becoming addicted after treatment. A whole number of new pain-killers chemically related to morphine were developed, and many were impressively effective; but although in the exuberance of discovery these were hailed as at last the pain-killers without risk of addiction—the risk in fact remained.

One of these promising new preparations was produced in 1898 by research chemists at a Bavarian dye-works, who were also applying a chemical variation of the morphine molecule. They established that the pain-reducing effect of the new substance was four to eight times stronger than that of morphine. They observed no indications for addiction risks. The hero in the fight against pain they jubilantly called 'heroin', and recommended the new drug to heal morphine addicts from their dependence.

These high hopes were followed by a terrible disappointment. Heroin, it proved, was an even more addictive drug than morphine; in fact it is the most dangerous addictive drug so far known. Luckily there are less harmful drugs today for most pain. But the danger of addiction seems to be inseparably linked with a substance's ability to reduce very severe pain.

Cocaine, the active substance in coca leaves, was isolated in 1860 by Albert Niemann, a chemist at Göttingen University. It was a long time before any other researchers took an interest in cocaine. One of the first, in the early 'eighties, was Sigmund Freud, who at that time had not thought of psychoanalysis. He hoped he could wean morphine addicts from their addiction through cocaine. 'This divine plant,' he wrote, 'which satisfies the hungry, strengthens the weak and makes them forget their misfortune . . . One feels an access of self-control, one feels more vigorous and able-bodied. . . .' Freud also talked of 'exhilaration and persistent euphoria, which is in no way to be distinguished from the normal euphoria of healthy people. . . . One is simply normal and soon finds it hard to believe one is under any outside influence. . . . It is completely without the sense of alteration which accompanies exhilaration through alcohol, and also without alcohol's unpleasant effects.'

Nowhere else in his many scientific works does Freud indulge in such extravagant raptures. They are to be found time and again in the statements of scientists about their first contacts with little-known psychoactive drugs. The pleasantness of brain manipulation seems to be so overwhelming that they lose all restraint and critical faculty and become enthusiastic proselytisers. Freud's subjective experiences were much too meagre, of course, to support such far-reaching assertions, but he was finally convinced of the rightness of his judgement. He sent cocaine to his fiancée, gave it to his sisters and praised it among friends and acquaintances. A colleague to whom he recommended cocaine as an antidote to morphine addiction became addicted to cocaine and died of it. 'In short,' writes his biographer Ernest Jones, 'from the standpoint of our present knowledge he was well on the way to becoming a danger to society.'

Neither Freud nor his fiancée turned into cocaine addicts, but sniffing cocaine became the fashion before the end of the 'eighties. A second wave of cocaine-taking started at the beginning of the First World War. It was very widespread in the 'twenties, although it had long become clear by then that, besides being euphoric, cocaine often produced fear and hallucinations. Collapses with fatal results after an overdose often occurred; and the addiction often ended in megalomania, persecution mania and complete madness. Today cocaine addiction is mainly a South American problem, where hundreds of thousands of Indians, perhaps even millions, still chew their beloved coca leaves. It should possibly be mentioned for the sake of the anxious that despite its name there is no cocaine in Coca-Cola!

Pain-killers, sleeping pills, amphetamines

Shortly before the end of the nineteenth century, German drug manufacturers presented the first synthetically produced psychoactive drugs: three pain-fighters which did not reduce agonising pain but could help with the less severe kind of pain. All three substances, acetyl-salicylic acid (first trade name: aspirin), phenacetin and aminophenazon (first trade name: pyramidon), are still extremely popular today. Against headache and toothache, slight rheumatic aches, pain during menstruation and with minor injuries—

chemists sell a large number of prescription-free drugs which contain at least one of the three substances. When doctors repeatedly complain about the widespread misuse of pain-killers, they are referring as a rule to these preparations easily accessible to everybody.

Today, sixty years after its introduction into medicine, acetyl-salicylic acid is the most used drug in the world. It is sold under dozens of brand names. Over twenty-five million pounds of it are produced a year by American manufacturers alone. All three substances are consumed in the United States and in Europe to an extent which causes serious doubts as to its correct usage. Many people swallow many pain-killer tablets every day throughout the year, with consequences ranging from permanent migraine to dangerous blood diseases and fatal kidney complaints.

The year 1903 started a new era in chemical brain manipulation: the great age of sleeping tablets began. With veronal the first narcotic based on barbituric acid came on to the market. In the course of time chemists succeeded in producing a large number of further barbiturates, of which some also acquired great importance as anaesthetics. But these chemical aids to slumber had two serious disadvantages: barbiturates, taken in excess, are highly poisonous (and therefore greatly favoured in suicide attempts), and they can become habit-forming and addictive. Barbiturate addicts take the sleeping tablets in the day as well, often in enormous quantities, and not all of them become tired or 'dopy' from doing so. Some addicts find the effect positively stimulating.

Meanwhile sleep-promoting substances were discovered, too, in a number of different classes of chemical. There are drugs which are less poisonous and also less addictive than the barbiturates. The triumph of a completely 'non-poisonous' sleeping tablet (no one could kill himself with it as with a barbiturate) led to the terrible tragedy of thalidomide. Probably this has taught society a lesson, so that sleeping tablets still on the market and those developed since then are more stringently watched for possible future side-effects. For all that, it does not seem very wise to put oneself to sleep regularly with one of these drugs, as millions of people do every night. Quite apart from other dangers, chemically induced sleep, it has been proved (see Chapter 18), is not of the same quality as natural sleep.

Wakefulness as well as sleep can be artificially induced. Coffee and tea, which contain caffein, have long been known for their stimulant effect: the cup that cheers, and also the cup that keeps you awake when you are very tired. Chemists have produced drugs called amphetamines which are far more potent than caffein in banishing sleep and exhaustion. The first amphetamine was synthesised in 1887, but it did not attract much interest for half a century. Then in 1936 psychologists began to test the effects of an amphetamine on students who had volunteered as guinea-pigs. They liked the effects, word got round, and soon students suffering from fatigue and staleness before exams were reaching for their amphetamine tablets.

In the Second World War amphetamines were given out to keep over-tired soldiers awake. In the 'sixties experts on drug poisoning noticed an increasing abuse of amphetamines, which a dynamic industry was producing as hard as it could. Many people became familiar with these drugs when they were fighting not fatigue but overweight: amphetamines reduce appetite. They were therefore offered as appetite-inhibitors; some of them still are.

Their effect depends on switching off the controls which normally protect a person from excessive fatigue. So they increase the body's efficiency at the time but they also give a feeling of heightened mental capacity. Thinking seems to be sharpened, reflexes seem quicker, powers of concentration improved. According to expert opinion this feeling is illusory. In any case the actual or supposed mental impetus does not last. Flights of imagination set in, and the attempt to compel the desired effect by increasing the dose only makes the disaster worse. It often leads to the amphetamine addict reaching a condition like schizophrenia. Amphetamines are of course far more dangerous than tea and coffee, which, taken in moderation by healthy people, can scarcely do any harm!

LSD

For five years the effect of this synthetically produced substance remained undiscovered. Then, another two decades later, in the early 'sixties, it gave rise to violent controversies.

In 1938, working for Sandoz, a pharmaceutical company in Basle, Albert Hoffmann synthesised a substance called d-lysergic acid-diethylamide, shortened to LSD. One day in April 1943, when he was working with LSD, he was overcome by a strange malaise, and felt no longer capable of continuing his chemical experiments. 'At home,' he reported later, 'I lay down and sank into a not unpleasant state like intoxication, characterised by extremely lively fantasy. In a semi-trance, with closed eyes, fantastic images of extraordinary vividness and with intensive kaleidoscopic colour-play were continually crowding in on me. After about two hours this condition passed off.' Hoffmann concluded that the LSD must have caused the hallucinating coma.

Psychiatrists and psychotherapists tried without notable success to make this hallucinogen useful to patients. The publicity media did not show any great interest in Hoffmann's discovery till 1961, when Timothy Leary, a psychology don at Harvard, made LSD 'trips' the centre of a new religion he now proclaimed. Suddenly, LSD hallucinations were the thing to have. Maximum efforts were made in illegal 'chemical labs' to meet the growing demand, while one state after another declared LSD a dangerous drug.

It is notable what an incredibly small dose of LSD is needed to produce very impressive hallucinations, whether pleasant or, with a bad trip, extremely alarming. A dose of .02 to .06 milligrams is enough. With a single gram of LSD a good 20,000 people could procure themselves hallucinations; with 3 kilograms (about 6½ lb.) all sixty million inhabitants of West Germany could be sent on a trip. No wonder that Hoffmann on his first close acquaintance with the hallucinogen was not at all conscious of having absorbed any.

That such a small amount of LSD can cause such drastic changes in brain activity seems all the more amazing in view of the fact that with mescalin, the hallucinogen agent in the peyote cactus, over ten thousand times the effective LSD dose is apparently required. And even more amazing still: only a fraction of the LSD, about a tenth, reaches the brain at all; the rest collects in liver and kidneys, to be then discharged.

Drugs for the mentally sick

For a long time every new psychoactive drug discovered set the doctors, especially the psychiatrists, extra problems. They found themselves in no position to release the many victims of alcohol from their fatal situation. Then came addicts of morphine, cocaine and heroin, the barbiturates and the amphetamines and finally distracted LSD-swallowers. The things completely missing were substances which did not put healthy brains in need of help, but helped to heal sick brains.

In 1952, when French researchers discovered the first drug with which the mentally sick could be effectively treated, a new era began in psychiatry. Within a few years a fundamental change took place in the life of psychiatric clinics and mental hospitals.

To start with, it was another of the famous accidental discoveries. Jean Delay and his colleagues in the drug company Rhône-Poulenc, doing research on the anti-histamines (antidotes to allergies like hay fever), developed chlorpromazine. It then turned out that chlorpromazine could suppress excitement states in patients with schizophrenia and manic conditions, and that it soon made the patients fully approachable again.

Until the introduction of chlorpromazine and a number of allied substances afterwards developed, which are collectively called analeptics, mental hospitals were predominantly institutions for long-term care and nursing. In them doctors and nurses protected the deranged from a hostile world—and protected the world from the deranged. But now clinics grew up where most mental patients could be effectively helped. A dark chapter in medicine, full of misunderstanding and helplessness, which only too often led to the most cruel treatment of the mentally ill, found its hopeful conclusion. The bars disappeared from many 'asylum' windows, the heavy locks from many doors. Most of the isolation cells, formerly designed for specially fractious patients, have long been converted into work-rooms or given some other unspecialised use.

Occupational therapy, though in principle pioneered earlier than the discovery of the analeptical drugs, did not reveal its full advantages until used in conjunction with them; for many patients the new drugs are needed to create the conditions for a positive occupational therapy. It is the same with psychotherapy and group therapy: many patients with mental disorders are not susceptible to these forms of treatment until they have received analeptics.

The most significant effect of the new drugs, however, is surely a change in the attitude of the healthy to their mentally sick fellow-beings. Slowly but irresistibly recognition is gaining ground that the mentally sick should not be treated as lepers, that they are not sinners, bear no guilt for their sickness and are not hopeless cases, but patients who can be healed. Like patients with physical complaints, they can be helped by doctors, so that they have good prospects of returning into the society of the healthy.

Still in the 'fifties, soon after the development of the analeptics, the first drugs were discovered for treating patients with depressions. Like the analeptics, the anti-depressants proved a therapeutic breakthrough in a field which had hitherto offered doctors few treatment possibilities. An impression of the extent of the problem is given by the estimate that a good one per cent of the population (six to seven hundred thousand people in West Germany) suffer from clinical depressions. This does not include those who are depressed from grief over a bereavement, an unhappy love affair, a drastic change for the worse in their material affairs, or similar anxieties and sadness. We may all suffer from such a depression periodically, and as its reason is recognisable, our reactions appear understandable to others. Special long-term medical treatment is generally not necessary.

It is quite different with the non-organic depressions which occur for no obvious reason. The depressive broods, finding no way out of his despair. He feels empty, incapable of decisions, a failure; he is tormented by anxiety and guilt feelings; suffers from insomnia and from aches and pains in various parts of his body; often he contemplates suicide. The picture can vary greatly, however, for every depressive patient has his own particular depression. So out of the two dozen or so substances which have meanwhile been adapted for fighting depression, it is important to find the one with the most favourable effect in each case.

For brain researchers the anti-depressants had a special interest because it was possible to make discoveries about their mode of action (see Chapter 14). Today there are well-based ideas on what disorders in the brain's metabolism lead to depressions and how anti-depressants affect the brain's chemical processes.

The 'fifties saw, finally, the discovery of a third group of important drugs for treating mental illnesses: the tranquillisers. The first of these, developed in the United States, was Meprobamate, which quickly became known all over the world under the trade name of Miltown. It proved a help towards achieving psychological balance even under great stress, damping down feelings of despair and fear, moderating uneasiness and nervous tensions, and also alleviating psychosomatic illnesses. No wonder that tranquillisers are today among the drugs most in demand; warnings against their abuse are unceasing. Meprobamate has long been superseded by new discoveries. Undisputed for years at the top of the tranquilliser league are two products of the Swiss firm Hoffmann-LaRoche, with names which bring hope to people in many countries who feel 'weary and heavy laden'. Millions look every day for the peace and calm they cannot create from their own resources, through librium and valium, household words which have become symbols of our time.

Ether

There are, of course, far more substances than those mentioned with which the brain's activity can be influenced and which are sometimes used for that purpose. Many of these drugs are exotic specialities of only local importance, but connoisseurs in Europe and America have been able to achieve interesting results from such improbable-sounding sources as nutmeg, various chemical solutions and ether.

To most people who have experienced it as an anaesthetic and do not remember it with any pleasure, a predilection for ether seems incomprehensible. But in the eighteen-thirties and forties ether parties were a craze in the United

States. One observant participant, Dr. Crawford Long, living in Jefferson, Georgia, noticed that those under its influence incurred injuries without complaining of pain; this led him to the discovery of ether as an anaesthetic. About the same time many Irishmen took ether, and towards the end of the century the taste was also acquired in Germany, especially East Prussia. In the town of Memel nearly thirty thousand gallons were sold in 1897 alone. As late as 1939 the authorities in one region felt obliged to make ether-drinking a criminal act. In other regions the 'Hoffmann drops', a mixture of three parts ether and one part alcohol, specially popular with women for decades, could only be sold on prescription.

What is the attraction in ether? Guy de Maupassant (who came into contact with it as patient, not as addict) describes it thus:

'The pain had vanished, melted away, dissolved. There was an enormous acuteness of understanding, a new way of seeing, judging, assessing things and life, with the complete confidence, the absolute certainty, that this way was the right one. And suddenly the old image from the Bible came into my mind: I felt as if I had eaten of the fruits of the tree of knowledge.'

Drugs and their dangers

To establish a clear order out of the bewildering number of substances which act upon the brain, scientists have put forward various systems. Jean Delay, for instance, to whom we owe the first drug for treating schizophrenics, suggested a division into three categories:

(1) Substances with a predominantly sedative effect (analeptics, tranquillisers, sleeping tablets, anaesthetics, pain-killers);

(2) Substances with predominantly stimulant effect (antidepressants, caffein, amphetamines, alcohol, morphine, heroin, cocaine);

(3) Substances which cause hallucinations (hashish, mescalin, LSD, belladonna and nightshade varieties, drugs in fly agaric and in Mexican fungi).

The action of the various drugs on the brain is so complex, however, that any system is about as satisfactory as categorising a row of peas by their size. Thus Delay puts alcohol and morphine among stimulants, although alcohol, which at first 'stimulates' by deadening the inhibitions, can induce sleep, as can morphine, which is also a pain-killer.

Where does tobacco come into this system? Its effect depends largely on the situation: it calms smokers when they are excited, and cheers them up when they are tired or despondent. Because of this contradictory effect many smokers react with embarrassment if asked what they actually get out of smoking. That it has its effect on the brain is obvious enough when heavy smokers try to stop. The affected regions of the brain revolt against this attempt, and even the awareness of the thinking part of the brain, that there is scarcely anything more dangerous for lungs, heart and circulation than cigarette smoke, is often not much lasting help.

Altogether the human brain finds it extraordinarily difficult to think and talk soberly about drugs, to weigh up their pleasant sides and their dangers and then act accordingly. The uncritical enthusiasm and minimising of dangers to health on the one side are often met by completely extravagant attacks on the other.

In Turkey, for instance, coffee-drinkers were once flogged, coffee-lovers had their tongues cut out, or those caught in the act of drinking coffee were sewn up in a sack and thrown into the sea. The same sort of fate befell coffee-lovers in Russia. Later on, some ingenious civil servant invented a coffee tax, after which the drinkers of this dangerous beverage had peace from the authorities. Yet at the end of the nineteenth century a respected pharmacologist could still write of the coffee-drinker: 'The sufferer trembles and loses his self-control. He looks pinched. As with other drugs, a new dose of the poison sometimes brings relief, but at the cost of future misery.' Of tea-drinkers it was said at the time: 'An hour or two after breakfast when tea has been drunk, the sufferer may be overcome by a depressing feeling of anxiety, so that talking is a great strain. Speech may become faint and indistinct, and through afflictions like these the best years of life may be ruined.'

The danger presented by these well-meaning but unfounded exaggerations is patent: even justified warnings about really dangerous drugs are no longer taken seriously. The present drug debate began in a very similar way. Hashish and heroin were often mentioned in one breath, and the illegal trade in both was prosecuted with the same intensity, although heroin is vastly more dangerous. While experts and laymen alike argue about the actual effects caused by the hemp products hashish and marihuana, and in what circles and circumstances these effects occur, it is established that heroin inevitably leads to decline and ruin on every front: moral, social, intellectual and physical. Only a few injections are enough to produce addiction. Six to seven years after the beginning of heroin addiction there is acute physical deterioration, though many addicts, of course, have developed liver complaints long before this, infecting themselves through unsterilised injections—and many will have already died of an overdose.

It would be a mistake to assume that they are ready to pay this price because the joys of paradise are beckoning them. Addicts have long ceased to enjoy their drug. It merely reduces the intolerable withdrawal symptoms which very quickly set in when they cannot obtain any heroin. Between the drug and substances in the brain, chemical processes are taking place which are naturally not subject to the will. The drug gets into the metabolism of the brain in such a way that the brain from then on finds it extremely difficult to live without the intruder.

The withdrawal symptoms are so appalling that even those looking after addicts are tempted to end their suffering with an injection of the drug. R. S. de Ropp has described the symptoms as follows:

'About twelve hours after the last dose of morphine or heroin, the addict becomes uneasy. A feeling of faintness comes over him, he yawns, shivers and sweats at the same time, while a watery fluid runs from his eyes and through his nose, which feels to him as if "hot water were running up into the mouth". For a few hours, tossing restlessly, he falls into an abnormal sleep which addicts call "greed sleep". On waking, 18 to 24 hours after taking the last dose, he enters the deeper regions of his "personal Hell". The yawning becomes so violent that he may dislocate his jaw. Thin mucus flows from the nose, tears pour from the eyes. The pupils are much enlarged, the skin itself is cold. . . .

His bowels begin to work with unprecedented force. The stomach walls contract in violent jerks and cause explosive vomiting, often with blood in the vomit. So violent are the contractions of the bowels that the body outside looks quite grooved and knotty, as if snakes were locked in battle under the skin. The fierce stomach pains increase rapidly. The bowels are continually emptied, so that there may be up to sixty watery stools a day.'

The Munich psychologist and drug expert Jürgen vom Scheidt, who quoted this description, completes it thus:

'Thirty-six hours after his last dose the addict is completely finished. In desperate efforts to alleviate the shivers racking his body, he puts on all the blankets he can find. The whole body is shaken with convulsions, and his feet make involuntary kicking movements, for which addicts have coined the macabre but extremely vivid expression "kicking the habit". Sleep and quiet are quite impossible during the withdrawal. The patient is continually tossed around by painful spasms of all the muscles in the body. Quite often he begins to let out appalling yells. Sometimes it happens that he writhes in his own vomit and excrement like a sick beast.'

A small dose of morphine or heroin is enough to assuage all the suffering in a moment. 'It is a dramatic experience,' writes the American drug expert Harris Bell, 'to observe how a wretched, pathetic individual, as soon as he has had an intravenous injection of some morphine, stands before you half an hour later, shaved, clean, laughing and joking.' Such an interruption of the withdrawal has of course the consequence that the agonies of withdrawal start again, normally passing off after about a week. At the end of the withdrawal cure the patient is completely exhausted, digestion and water metabolism are still disturbed. The danger of his succumbing to the drug again remains great.

Alcohol

Clearly, rigorous defence measures against heroin are completely justified. If, however, the consequences of heroin are compared with those of alcohol, the latter proves a far more serious health problem. More impressively than any other example, the relation of our society to alcohol demonstrates the irrational nature of human behaviour over drugs.

According to an American estimate for 1970, about four thousand people in the United States died of other drugs than alcohol, especially heroin. About ten times that number succumbed to alcohol in the same year, not counting accidental victims (and about 400,000 people brought themselves to premature death through cigarettes). In West Germany alone there are today at least 600,000 alcoholics in need of treatment, and possibly considerably more than that.* The number of alcoholics all over the world in need of treatment is estimated at twenty million.

But alcoholism is a disease from which not only the drinker himself suffers. This is, of course, true also of heroin and other addictive drugs; but heroin addicts are mainly young people without families, whereas a great many alcoholics are adults with a wife or husband and often young children, who will scarcely grow up without traumatic effects from their parent's repulsive complaint. Then again, a third of the traffic accidents are caused by alcohol, and a large proportion, two-thirds in the United States, of all offences committed are connected with alcohol. It does not need much insight to recognise that human society would be better off without it.

Yet while heroin is rightly under a strict ban, alcohol can be bought almost without restrictions, and what is more, the producers of alcoholic drinks can unhindered use all their energies to increasing alcohol consumption through expensive and suggestive advertising. They can do this, of course, only because the majority of those addressed find the effect of alcohol pleasant.

No other means of brain manipulation is so closely bound up with ordinary life and special occasions, with the high points and low points of human life. Every joyful or sad event, cold or heat, solitude or company, inhibitions or relaxation, work or leisure, too much money or too little—

---

* Translator's Note: According to Dr. Henry Miller, in *Medicine and Society* (August 1973), of all the drugs used in Britain for non-medical purposes alcohol and tobacco are by far the most dangerous to health. There are over 350,000 chronic alcoholics, with a suicide rate 80 times the normal, and alcohol plays a part in at least two-thirds of the crimes committed in this country. We smoke 350 million cigarettes a day and this causes over 40,000 deaths and contributes to at least another 150,000 annually. There are fewer than 300 heroin addicts in Britain.

all may be causes for drinking. Our brain, in fact, will find almost any excuse for exposing itself to alcohol.

Reckoning the amount of alcohol consumed annually in West Germany in the form of beer and wine, spirits and liqueurs, we reach an amount of well over two gallons per person; and the average is obviously much higher taking into account small children and teetotallers. Even two gallons is quite a lot of drink, the content of about 36 bottles of spirits, 150 bottles of wine or 900 bottles of beer. The same citizens whose union representatives fear for their social welfare when wage increases do not greatly outweigh loss of purchasing power, will cheerfully spend hundreds of marks per person a year on alcoholic drinks. In 1969 twenty million marks, far too small a sum, were available for education, while the inhabitants allocated thirty thousand million to alcohol and tobacco alone. Similar statistics could be given for most other affluent countries.

Even drinkers who cannot be accused of addiction are irrational on the subject. The prospect of having to give up alcohol's pleasure-giving stimulation scares people so much that their brain is incapable of considering the matter 'soberly'.

Attempts have of course been made at prohibition: for instance in Finland in 1919 and in the United States in 1920. The experiments begun so hopefully ended in a fiasco. A lively smuggling trade developed, becoming in America the basis for gangsterism. Alcoholism did not diminish, and the danger to health grew through the impurity of the illicit alcohol.

An apparent paradox: alcohol is rendered specially dangerous just because only a proportion of the people who drink regularly or often become addicted. Opium and morphine, heroin and cocaine lead much more rapidly to addiction, and their victims go much faster downhill. But the dire effects keep most people from getting involved with these drugs at all. The preponderance of enemies and of the indifferent makes it possible to prescribe these hard drugs and keep within bounds transgressions of the ban. A ban on alcohol, on the other hand, cannot be enforced. Those in danger remain completely unprotected. A publicly sanctioned means of addiction lures them to their sickness.

12

The Nerve Cells

It is understandable that the spectacular and uncanny experiments with brain stimulation should have been recognised as decisive advances in brain research. Even though many of the discoveries were made on the brains of animals, they have indeed added immensely to our knowledge about the human brain. But these discoveries and those gained from split brains do little towards explaining how the brain actually functions, what principles it works on, what makes it capable of its incomparable achievements, which seem all the more fantastic the more one learns about them. And what happens when a psychoactive drug influences the brain? What chemical processes take place between the drug and the substances of the brain? Why can these processes influence the brain's activity so extensively? Before researchers succeeded in answering these questions, they had to find out what exactly was meant by terms like 'brain activity'.

With the experiments described so far, normal brain activity was more or less drastically disturbed. Researchers and doctors inserted electrical current, severed natural connections, removed selected areas of the brain, or simply observed the consequences of disorders deriving from sickness processes or injuries. They did what an adventurous do-it-yourself mechanic might do, when confronting a complicated technical apparatus with a structure he does not understand: he snips through a wire here, breaks contact there, and watches what happens.

It is easier for him; he can see clearly what he is dealing with. The brain researcher, on the other hand, stimulating parts deep in the brain's interior, sticks the electrodes into a gelatinous mass. Precision based on previous experience, and sometimes 'a little bit of luck', help him to hit particular points at which he is aiming. But what actually happens in the brain when a particular stimulus at a particular point produces a particular reaction remains obscure with this sort of experiment. The brain reacts, but does not surrender its secret.

Other methods of investigation have made further progress: neuroanatomists, neurophysiologists and neurochemists have succeeded in revealing amazing details about the brain's precision structure and mode of action. The brain has repeatedly proved a quarry for discoveries worthy of the Nobel Prize.

Tubes and balls

The first discoveries were made, of course, long before there was a Nobel Prize. Early anatomists could see with the naked eye that the brain consisted of grey and white matter. After the invention of the microscope, researchers also inspected brain tissue with these at first very imperfect magnifiers.

In 1684 Anton van Leeuwenhoek, a Dutch business man who was one of the founders of scientific microscopy, discovered in the white matter 'tubes' which were really nerve fibres. But this discovery and similar observations of other researchers were rejected as illusory by 'experts' who were obviously less skilled in the use of a microscope. In 1791, for instance, the otherwise distinguished Mainz anatomist S. T. von Soemmering wrote that 'under the magnifying glass both the grey and the marrowy part of the brain mass appear as tough, sticky, inert, small lumps or balls, rather transparently sticking together'.

Science did not officially recognise the nerve fibres until 1816, when G. R. Treviranus, a Bremen natural scientist, gave an exact description of the 'nerve tubes'. In 1833 another German biologist, C. G. Ehrenburg in Berlin, saw nerve cells also under the microscope. In the ganglia of the spinal cord nerves of birds he observed 'very large, almost ball-shaped irregular bodies forming the actual swellings, which are more like a gland substance'. He did not guess, however, what he had discovered.

But the next steps followed quickly. The Czech physiologist J. E. Purkinje reported in 1837 that the nerve balls, which he called 'ganglia bodies', had different shapes in the different areas of the brain, that they had prolongations and a nucleus. Two years later Theodor Schwann in Louvain, founder of the doctrine that living things were made up of cells, expressed his conviction that the nerve balls were 'nerve cells'; and again a year later Adolf Hannover found 'it more than probably that the brain fibres derive from the brain cells'.

There was still argument about it. But more and more researchers after detailed microscopic studies drew the conclusion that nerve cells and nerve fibres were not the different elements in the nervous system, but that the nerve fibres were parts of the nerve cells. The first realistic picture of a nerve cell, drawn from microscopic investigation, was found at Bonn in the papers of a young don called Otto Deiters who died of typhoid in 1863 when he was only twenty-nine. His professor published his work two years later.

The drawing made by Deiters over a century ago still

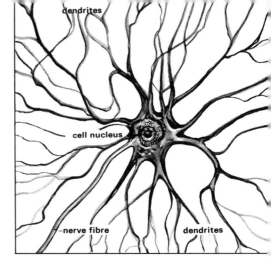

Nerve cells are strange structures. The German researcher Otto Deiters was the first to achieve, over a century ago, a realistic idea of a nerve cell with its long appendages. The drawing shown here has been made on the model of Deiters's picture.

looks amazingly modern. It shows a strange structure: a cell with a relatively large nucleus, surrounded by dark-coloured cell plasma; but striking especially for its long, hair-thin branches. 'Hair-thin' is not to be taken literally; in reality the plasma threads are often only the hundredth of a millimetre thick and so are much thinner than hair. No other cell in the organism has such plasma threads.

These threads with their many branches are today called dendrites (from the Greek word *dendron*=tree). At one point, however, a special extension comes out of the nucleus just as thin as the dendrites but smooth-walled and, so far as the drawing reaches, with no branches. Deiters recognised correctly that a nerve cell has many dendrites but only one nerve fibre.

Anatomy of a nerve cell

On all three sections of a nerve cell, cell body, dendrites and nerve fibre, researchers have revealed far more than Deiters could then know.

The cell body contains not only all the structures indispensable for the metabolism of a normal cell; it is crammed full of component parts. Its power stations are very small bodies called mitochondria (from the Greek words *mitos* and *khondros* = thread cartilages), and it probably has even more of these than liver cells, which show a particularly intensive metabolism. Small granules called ribosomes, the cell's protein factories, are so thickly packed in the nerve cell that they give the cell body its dark colouring.

The energy produced by the mitochondria is responsible, as neurochemists have shown, for an immense production of proteins. The Zurich neurophysiologist Konrad Akert speaks of 'incredibly large turnover figures for protein'. A nerve cell, so scientists have calculated, synthesises fifteen thousand protein molecules a second. Akert calls this protein production 'glandlike'. So it is an essential function of the nerve cells to produce masses of protein, but what is all the protein for? An obvious question, to which there is so far no clear answer, only hypotheses, for instance that the protein may be needed for the functioning of memory.

Power stations and factories (mitochondria and ribosomes) are less close together in the dendrites, and they become more sparse the further the region under examination is from the cell body. In the plasma of the nerve fibre there are only a few distinguishable structures but it is just this part of the nerve cell which is most striking. It is often surrounded by a many-layered covering of fatty substances and protein— the myelin—which has a white gleam. This is why areas in the brain and the spinal cord, which consist predominantly of nerve fibres, look to be 'white matter'. Close inspection shows that the white myelin does not cover the nerve fibre to a uniform thickness, but is broken up every one or two millimetres by a ring-shaped node. At the node the nerve fibre is uncovered.

Considering how thin a nerve fibre is, about a hundredth

This drawing makes concrete the size relationship between the cell body of a nerve cell and a nerve fibre several inches long. The ellipse above represents the much magnified cell body from which the nerve fibre extends.

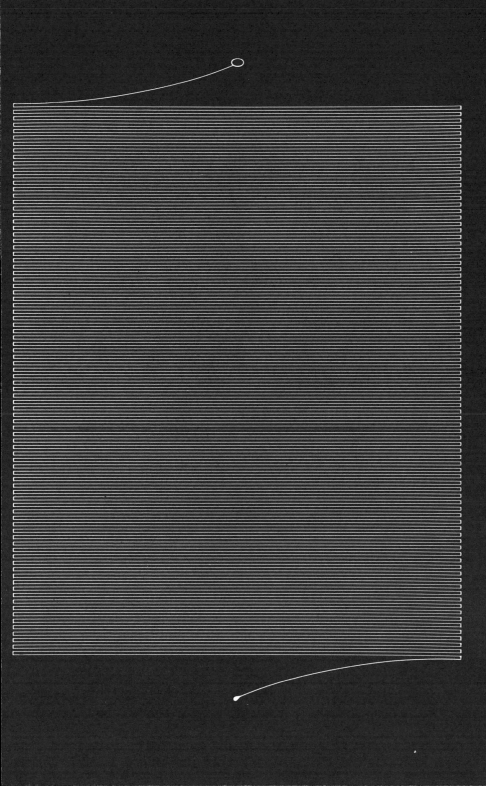

of a millimetre, it seems incredible that such a cell appendage can become over a yard long in man's spinal cord and even longer with giraffes and elephants.

The length of nerve fibres may reach many thousand times their thickness. The nerve fibres of brain cells are a good deal shorter. But in the spinal cord as in the brain the nerve fibre usually splits up into many branches in the part furthest from the cell body.

What Deiters had recognised in laborious microscopic studies became plainly visible in 1875 for anyone who wished to see nerve cells. In that year Camillo Golgi, then a doctor in a small town near Milan, reported on a method which made it much easier to investigate the nervous system. He treated sections of nerve tissue first with potassium bichromate, then with silver nitrate: this made fibres and dendrites show up in black even in the thinnest branches, while the surrounding tissue remained uncoloured.

Neurones or network?

It was now clearly recognisable that the nerve cells formed a plexus of complex ramifications, but fine as these preparations were, they did not prove good enough to prevent a scientific dispute which lasted for decades. The most intensive examination under the best microscope did not reveal whether the nerve cells only touched each other through their thin extensions or whether they formed a network by which one cell passed directly into another.

The former view was called the theory of neurones, the term used by doctors for the whole nerve cell including dendrites and fibre. 'The nervous system', declared the German scientist Wilhelm Waldeyer, 'consists of many anatomically and genetically independent nerve units (neurones).' One of the supporters of this theory was the Spanish anatomist Santiago Ramon y Cajal, for a long time the most famous of all brain researchers. With the aid of the colouring method developed by Golgi, he studied all parts of the nervous system, and there are an immense number of findings with which his name is associated. In the dispute over the theory of neurones Golgi was on the other side, believing in a continuous network of nerves; it was reported that he was so embittered that he refused to receive a visit from Cajal. The Nobel Prize Committee, ignoring the controversy, awarded the Prize for medicine to both men, 'in recognition of their work on the structure of the nervous system'.

The controversy lasted, with new protagonists, until the 'fifties. Through the electronic microscope and investigations whereby individual nerve cells could be monitored, it was finally settled in favour of the theory of neurones. This was the only way in which the nervous system could function at all (see next chapter).

Nerve cells with their dendrites and fibres are very extended structures, so there must be something else to fill out the brain. Besides the ten to fifteen thousand million nerve cells, the brain contains about ten times as many cells which are not nerve cells. These 'glia cells' (from the Greek word for glue) look less exciting, and for a long time they were regarded merely as gap-fillers. They are certainly more than this, and some of their functions have since been discovered, while others are so far only hypotheses.

Glia cells certainly provide the nerve cells with raw material needed for the intensive metabolic processes. They establish connections between blood vessels and nerve cells. Particular glia cells produce gleaming white covers for nerve fibres. But many researchers believe there is evidence for glia cells being far more closely involved with the brain's activity than has hitherto been thought: for instance, they may be concerned with the information store which we prize as memory.

It is perhaps a pity that generations of brain researchers

rather neglected the glia cells, although there are so many more of them than nerve cells. But the enormous amount of research devoted to nerve cells has certainly been very rewarding. For today we not only know the structure of the neurones down to the finest detail; we are well informed on their mode of action.

13

The Transmitting of Electrical Signals

It is common knowledge that electricity plays an important part in the activity of the nerve cells or neurones. But that does not say much, considering the fineness of the nerve cells and the variety of the brain's functions which we all experience every day. Where does the electric current flow from and to? What size and speed does it have? After decades of investigations brain researchers today can answer such questions exactly; and they have discovered connection points between the nerve cells which have astonishing capacities.

Luigi Galvani, an anatomist in Bologna, is often called the discoverer of 'animal electricity', and he claimed himself to have discovered it. The story of how he got the idea in 1786 from the twitching of a frog's thigh is one of the few widely known stories in scientific history. In fact animal electricity had been proved before these observations, which anyhow Galvani fundamentally misinterpreted.

At the end of the seventeenth century scientists believed that the body's warmth was produced by the blood flowing into the veins. Since friction can produce both warmth and electricity, it was considered possible half a century later that electricity too came into the blood-vessels in this way. From blood-vessels to nerves was only a step: if (as was then thought, without any evidence) the nerves were narrow channels in which a nerve sap circulated, why should there not be electricity there too? It turned out that electrifying machines could make paralysed muscles twitch. But the electricity which produced these effects was applied from outside, whereas in 1772 actual animal electricity was proved from the study of electric fishes.

Electricity was soon the 'in' word. In Lyon in 1777 a scientific prize questionnaire asked: 'Which are the illnesses which depend on the smaller or larger quantity of electric fluid in the human body; and which are the remedies for each?' We need not go into the answers which won the prize in 1779.

In 1786 Galvani made his famous observation—although in one of the various versions of the story it was his wife who first saw the frog's thigh twitch. Anyhow, dead frogs were hanging on brass hooks on the balcony; their thighs were destined for experiments, food or both. Galvani had drawn the hooks through the frog's spinal cords. It was windy, so that the frogs swung to and fro on their hooks. Now and again they knocked against the iron rail of the balcony. Whenever they did so, it happened: the thigh twitched.

Galvani was convinced he had found the animal electricity on which there had been so much speculation at the time, and he was very ready to interpret his observations: 'We believe, therefore, that the (electric) fluid is made by the power of the brain and probably developed out of the blood.' But the crucial thing in Galvani's experimental dispositions, as Alessandro Volta proved soon afterwards, was certainly not the frog. Admittedly a current flowed, which made the thigh twitch, but it was caused by the fact that brass hook and iron rail were connected with each other; the frog was only the conductor. Galvani had discovered metal electricity, a discovery of no less significance, but one which did not interest him.

Animal electricity remained a disputed matter. It was not till the eighteen forties, when more sensitive measuring instruments had been constructed, that Emil Du Bois-Reymond in Berlin succeeded in proving that nerves did not merely conduct electric current passively; that their activity was connected with the continual production of electricity. In 1850 the versatile German physiologist and physicist Hermann von Helmholtz measured the speed at which an electrical signal was transmitted in the nerve: 27.25 metres (about ninety feet) a second, or—working by car speeds—about sixty m.p.h.

The measurement was accurate, but today we know that the transmission speed of a nerve signal may be less than $2\frac{1}{2}$ and more than 200 m.p.h. Whether a nerve signal creeps along like a leisurely stroller or shoots off at above the speed of a racing car, depends on the diameter of the nerve fibre concerned and on its insulation.

Somewhere round the time when Du Bois-Reymond and Helmholtz made their pioneering discoveries, the anatomists, too, had achieved remarkable results. The idea of a connection between the cells observed in the brain and the nerve fibres had become increasingly likely. These advances in anatomy and physiology created a solid basis from which nerve researchers could start gradually clarifying in more and more detail the way the nerve cells worked. Generations of scientists were concerned with this, including a dozen Nobel prize-winners: Sir Charles Scott Sherrington and Edward Douglas Adrian (both Great Britain), 1932; Otto Loewi (Austria) and Sir Henry Mallett Dale (Great Britain), 1936; Joseph Erlanger and Herbert Spencer Gasser (both United States), 1944; Sir John Eccles (Australia), Andrew Fielding Huxley and Alan Lloyd Hodgkin (both Great Britain), 1963; Ulf von Euler (Sweden), Julius Axelrod (United States), Sir Bernard Katz (Great Britain), 1970.

Despite their work there are still secrets so far unrevealed, but at least we know a great deal more today about the activity of the nerve cells.

Resting potential and action potential

Every nerve cell is part of a communications system which has connections stretching through the body, and which itself has a closely-meshed network of connections. It is an obvious idea that the nervous system works like a telephone network. But the transmission of information in the animal and in the human organism is quite a different process, it has been shown, from telephonic communications.

A communications technician can see at a glance that nerve cells with their nerve fibres are no use for 'telephoning'. The resistance offered to electric current by the viscous interior of a nerve fibre is about a hundred million times greater than in a copper wire. Moreover, the covering of a nerve fibre is not remotely comparable with the insulation of a good cable. Consequently an impulse transmitted from a source of current into a nerve fibre is immensely weakened after only a few millimetres.

Neurophysiologists like to compare the mechanism of information transmission in a nerve cell with the conducting principle of a fuse, at which the flame from one end goes along to the other. But besides the greater speed of the nerve signal, there is another crucial distinction in this analogy: the fuse cannot be used a second time when the flame has reached the end; whereas with a nerve cell every area which has passed on a signal is already prepared for a new signal a thousandth of a second later. Finally, electricity plays a decisive rôle in the nerve cell, while the burning down of a fuse has nothing to do with current.

Even in a state of rest, when a nerve cell is not transmitting any signal, there is a difference in electrical potential (voltage) between the inside and outside of the cell as between the two poles of a torch battery. The voltage could be measured with sensitive instruments; it is about seventy millivolts. The outside of the cell is the positive pole, the inside the negative. So to be accurate we should say that the voltage in the cell, referring to the outer side, is minus seventy millivolts. This voltage, since it was measured in the nerve cell's state of rest, is called rest voltage or resting potential.

The potential changes abruptly to the so-called action potential when a signal comes in and has to be transmitted. Scientists can simulate the situation for their investigations by tapping a nerve cell with an extremely thin wire connected to a source of current, and then giving the cell a slight electric shock. The voltage drops at once. On the oscilloscope, a device which shows on a screen how electric potentials change over time, a curve rises steeply from the -70 millivolt line to the resting potential. It reaches the zero line, goes a good bit past this, then drops again. The graph shows that the voltage returns for a short time, so long as the curve is above the zero line. During that time the inside forms the positive pole, the outside negative.

To test the nerve cell's reaction, researchers stimulated it with currents of various strengths, which produced a remarkable result: under a certain level the cell did not react with an action potential. Once this level, called the stimulation threshold, was passed, the curve went always to the same height, no matter how strong the current was. So nerve cells function according to an 'all-or-nothing' law. A stimulus which is not strong enough is ignored. In view of the vast number of stimuli to which a nerve cell in the organism is constantly exposed, this is certainly a very useful indifference.

What we have just considered was the reaction of a particular point in the nerve cell at the moment when a signal comes in. But the signal does not remain at this point, it is transmitted onwards. The change in voltage is infectious.

And when this process was investigated more closely, there was again a surprise: although nerve cells are relatively poor conductors with only moderate insulation, the signal runs on over longish stretches completely unimpaired. This raises the question of how such a thing is possible and what processes are responsible for the changes in electric potential. This, too, has been discovered by neurophysiologists.

Migrants at the cell membranes

The decisive processes take place in the fine membrane surrounding the inside of the nerve cell. Although only a hundredth of a millimetre thick, this not only holds the cell plasma together; it also lets a lot of it through. We must now see what it lets through and under what circumstances.

For the problem of nerve conducting, two of the many substances which may slip through the membrane are of special interest: potassium and sodium. Both are to be found in relatively large quantities in our food (sodium is a component of salt). Each of these potassium and sodium parts carries a simple positive charge. As with other electrically charged atoms or molecules, scientists speak of 'ions' (from the Greek word for going, travelling: ions in an electrical field travel to one of the poles in the field because of their charge).

Potassium and sodium ions are not regularly distributed in the nerve cells and their surroundings. Potassium ions are concentrated inside the cells, sodium ions outside. Since both kinds have a positive charge, this might lead to a neutralisation of the positive ions inside and outside. But the membrane does not let through both kinds of ions with the same readiness. Potassium ions can slip out far more easily than sodium ions can push in.

If that were to go on indefinitely, the inside of the cell would soon be very poor in potassium ions. But that con-

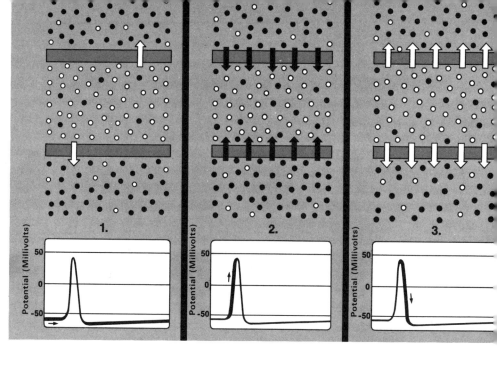

Brain researchers have been able to find out what happens in the nerve fibre when it transmits an electrical signal. In the inside of the fibre (between the grey beams) potassium ions (white circles) are in the majority; outside, sodium ions (black circles). In the resting state (left) the cell membranes are somewhat porous to potassium, but not to sodium. Inside the cell a deficit in positive electrical charge is therefore produced. When an electrical signal comes in, which has to be transmitted, the porousness of the cell membrane to sodium changes abruptly, so that inside the cell an excess of charge suddenly occurs (centre). Shortly afterwards the membrane closes to sodium and opens to potassium (right). The ion pump ensures the correct distribution of potassium and sodium ions: potassium inside, sodium outside. The resting potential is restored.

dition is avoided. A mechanism about which nerve researchers still know scarcely anything, and which for the moment they have called ion pump, ensures that 'deserting' potassium ions are pumped back into the cell and sodium ions are helped out. The pump, however, cannot completely stop the emigration of the potassium ions. Inside the cell some positive charge is always lacking. The inside of the membrane, compared with the outside, has a negative charge. This is what causes the resting potential.

When the nerve cell is stimulated, the porousness of the membrane to sodium suddenly changes. The ions held back will then flow in large numbers into the cell. Their positive charges make the negative resting potential turn into a positive action potential.

But this process is self-limiting. When a certain potential is reached, the membrane closes for sodium and opens for potassium. Crowds of potassium ions pour out, setting up a deficit again in positive charges: the resting potential. The ion pump ensures that the ions are soon correctly distributed again, potassium inside, sodium outside. The whole process from the replacement of rest potential by action potential to the restoration of the resting potential lasts about a thousandth of a second.

The ion pump is in constant need of energy. To produce it is no problem for the healthy and normally fed organism. Nerve signals, despite their unsatisfactory conductivity (from the standpoint of the communications technician), can thus be transmitted over long stretches without loss of information. The difference from a telephone is clear: in the nerve cell, it is not electric current which is primarily transmitted, but a wave of activity which is quickly passed on and is accompanied by a change of potential. It is in this sense that neurophysiologists talk about the fuse principle.

Assistance from squid

Seeing how long it took researchers to recognise nerve cells at all with the microscope, it may be asked how it was possible to discover the behaviour of the nerve cells in such fine detail. A justified question. Who knows with what modest knowledge we should have to be content without certain natural phenomena which nerve researchers have found extremely useful: giant nerve fibres.

Many lower animal species such as the squid have specially thick nerve fibres: these may be up to a millimetre thick, as against only a hundredth of a millimetre for human nerve fibres. Skilful physiologists have done a great deal with squid nerve fibres: for instance, they have stuck micro-electrodes into them to measure exactly the differences in potential between inside and outside; they have altered the composition of the fluid which washes around them; with the aid of a glass cannula thrust into the inside of the fibres they have tested the effect of different substances on the cell content.

Finally they even succeeded in squeezing out the cell content of the fibres like toothpaste from a tube and replacing it by injecting different chemical solutions into them. These interferences, which the giant nerve fibres proved strong enough to stand, made it possible to register the reactions of the membrane in the most varied circumstances and thereby to gain a picture of the processes which normally take place in it.

We owe most of the discoveries about the nerve cell's activity achieved through the giant nerve fibres of squid, to the British scientists Alan Lloyd Hodgkin and Andrew Fielding Huxley. In 1963, when they were awarded the Nobel Prize, they had been concerned with the giant fibres for twenty-four years. For a long time they were together at Cambridge, while the squid were at Plymouth, two hundred miles away. They devoted themselves so zealously to their studies on the coast that their wives complained of being 'squidows'.

But do their findings apply to the nerve cells of higher animals and especially man? This too has been investigated, and it appears that they are generally valid for all nerve cells. Nerve fibres have, however, been improved in the courses of evolution. Squid do not have the insulating cover to the fibres, the white myelin; this is only to be found in vertebrates. The processes at the membrane are basically the same, except for one difference: they take place with the covered nerve fibres only at the nodes where the membrane is exposed. Consequently the action potential does not glide continuously along the fibres but jumps from node to node. This allows a high transmission speed to be reached in man's thin nerve-fibres. The fibres with a myelin cover also work more economically.

So far we have only talked of what happens in the individual nerve cell. But a signal comes from somewhere, and it is transmitted forward over the cell border. The individual nerve cell is only a component of a comprehensive communications system. Simple as the principle seems whereby action potentials are conducted along the nerve fibres, the crossing of the border with good reason shows a great refinement of organisation. In the last years investigations of this have founded a special discipline: synaptology.

The vital synapses

'Synapse' (from the Greek word for connection) is the term used by neurophysiologists for the place where two nerve cells meet; or, more exactly, the contact of one end of the nerve fibre, mostly much ramified, with the cell body or a dendrite of another nerve cell. In the brain there are far more synapses than nerve cells. A nerve cell may be connected by synapses with up to ten thousand other nerve cells. Experts have reckoned that the billions of connections between the millions of nerve cells in a single human brain would extend to some 200,000–250,000 miles, the distance from the earth to the moon.

The scientists like Golgi who thought that the nervous system was a continuous network of cells cannot have had much concrete idea, we can say with hindsight, of how nerve signals find their way. In such a network the electrical impulses would have to wander around aimlessly. Instead of speeding to their destination by a practical path, they would spread out into any corners of the system. Without synapses it is hard to imagine how the connection arrangements essential for the functioning of the brain and the whole nervous system could be realised.

As we have seen, however, the controversy over the neurone theory was finally settled in the 'fifties when efficient electron microscopes made it possible to obtain a clear picture of the contact connection points. And then it transpired that nerve cells were separated from each other at every contact point not only by their membrane but also by a tiny gap. It is little more than a hundred thousandth of a millimetre, but wide enough to stop a nerve signal crossing it easily.

In order to cross, the electrical signal must be turned for the moment into a chemical one. This would seem to make the communication of information unnecessarily hard, but on closer view proves very practical. The required substance to help the signal over the gap is only stored on one side. As a result signals can only cross the gap in one direction. So a synapse works like a valve ensuring one-way traffic in the nerve cells. Action potentials always travel from the cell body to the ends of the nerve fibres, never the other way round.

Electron microscopes show clearly the three parts of a synapse: an end of a nerve fibre, which is slightly enlarged and is called a terminal bouton, the surface of the adjoining cell, and the gap between. In the terminal bouton a large number of small vesicles can be recognised, thicker than the gap is wide. They contain the transmitter substance. There are also a great many mitochondria (i.e. the power factories) in the bouton. On the other side of the gap there are no vesicles and not very many mitochondria.

The electron microscope photographs do not show what goes through the synapse when information is communi-

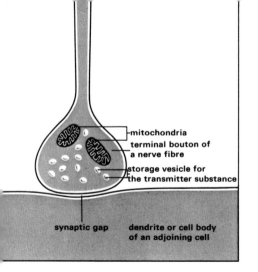

mitochondria

terminal bouton of
a nerve fibre

storage vesicle for
the transmitter substance

synaptic gap

dendrite or cell body
of an adjoining cell

*The transmission of a signal from
one nerve cell to another is very
finely regulated. When an
electrical signal has reached the
terminal bouton of a nerve fibre,
to cross the synaptic gap it has to
be transformed temporarily into a
chemical signal. The supply of
transmitter substance in the
storage vesicles is used for this.
Such an apparently complicated
procedure ensures that signals are
only transmitted in one direction.*

cated. But experiments with microelectrodes, partly again
on squid (which have giant synapses as well as giant nerve
fibres) and also chemical investigations, have thrown
considerable light on the processes at the gap.

An action potential which has arrived in the bouton comes
to an abrupt halt there. But before it dies away, it impels
some vesicles to pour transmitter substance into the synaptic
gap. The molecules cross the gap and on the other side meet
a membrane which is at the rest potential. Now the transmitter substance causes the same process as the one which
takes place in the nerve fibre under the influence of an
approaching action potential: the porousness of the membrane changes, first to sodium, then to potassium, and
finally the ion pump comes into action. On the other side
of the synaptic gap an action potential has again come into
being, which travels to the nerve fibre.

How the transmitter substance alters the porousness of
the membrane has not yet been satisfactorily explained. It
is certain, however, that the transmitter must quickly
disappear again from the gap. This can happen in various
ways, depending what the substance is: either the molecules
of the transmitter substance are directed back into the terminal bouton, or they are so far destroyed by enzymes that

they can no longer influence the membrane. In the latter case the problem arises that the destroyers must in turn be removed as quickly as possible from the gap. How this happens, like many other details, is still unknown.

It is only one of the functions of the synapses to act as valves regulating the flow of signals in the nervous system. The other function comes about from the fact that besides the synapses just described there is another kind which has exactly the opposite effect: instead of building an action potential again on the far side of the gap, these synapses reduce the capacity of the adjoining cell to be excited. In contrast to the 'exciting' synapses, they are called 'inhibiting' synapses. The same thing happens with them at first as with the exciting synapses: the action potential coming in sends a transmitter substance into the gap. But this substance does not first reduce the porousness to sodium ions which might invade the cell, but to potassium ions, which now stream out of it. The positive charge inside the cell is thereby reduced even more, while the negative charge on the outside increases. So for reaction on the 'all-or-nothing' principle, it needs an even stronger impulse than usual to produce an electric signal. An inhibiting synapse makes the stimulus threshold higher in the adjoining cell.

Is there a purpose in that? Inhibiting synapses, neurophysiologists assure us, are no less important than exciting ones. They immensely expand the connection possibilities in the brain. Every nerve cell, as has been said, is connected by synapses with thousands of other nerve cells, some of which transmit exciting and others inhibiting signals (though a particular nerve cell at its greatly ramified nerve fibre has only one kind of output from its terminal bouton: either only exciting or only inhibiting). At every moment a large number of exciting and inhibiting impulses hit the membrane. The nerve cell thus bombarded is constantly striking a balance, and according to which impulses are preponderant, the exciting or the inhibiting, an action potential is

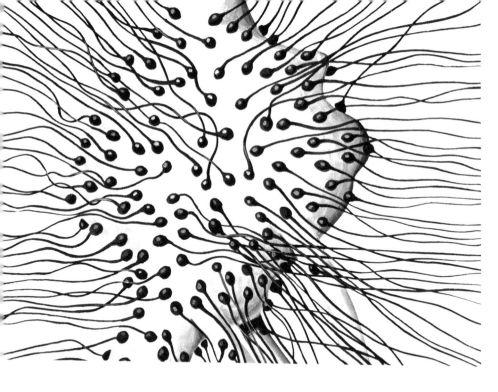

Each nerve cell is connected with thousands of others. Tightly packed on the surface of the nerve cell are the terminal boutons, the enlarged ends of finely branched nerve fibres.

either transmitted to the nerve fibre or it is not. Each of the thousand million nerve cells is thus a tiny calculating machine which adds and subtracts.

The electron microscope photograph will show whether a synapse represented is of the exciting or the inhibiting kind. The two kinds are distinguished certainly, however, in the transmitter substance.

In their efforts to discover what the tiny vesicles in the terminal boutons are filled with, synaptologists have achieved considerable success. But how do you analyse the content of vesicles which can scarcely be recognised even when magnified thirty thousand times?

A solution proved possible through a process whereby

brain tissue was first thoroughly broken up in a mixer. Then the flabby pulp was whirled round at a very high speed. The higher the number of revolutions, the finer the particles which sank to the bottom of the centrifuge container. Finally, as the electron microscope showed, in a fractionation achieved at a particularly high speed, the tiny terminal boutons were finally strongly concentrated. They had survived this harsh procedure unharmed. The point of this operation was to trace the action of the substances which might be active.

We know today that some act as transmitter substances in different parts of the nervous system. For instance gamma-amino-butyric acid and glycin act as inhibitors, acetylcholine and glutamic acid, noradrenalin and serotonin as exciters. Other substances spread over the brain are thought to be active also in the synapses.

More important for the layman than these mostly very complicated names is a basic discovery: satisfactory functioning of body and mind depends on the chemical processes in the synaptic gap continuing undisturbed in finely balanced equilibrium. If the action of a transmitter substance is inhibited or the destruction of the transmitter molecule is prevented after its work at the membrane is complete, there is a likelihood of severe damage to health or even death.

The deadly effect of the pesticide E 605, for instance, depends on a disturbance in the chemistry of the synapses. It blocks a substance called acetylcholine-esterase, which has the function of making the transmitter acetylcholine ineffective in the synaptic gap. Consequently, the membrane in the receiving nerve cell remains porous. No resting potential can now appear. The flow of information is so drastically disturbed that death ensues. The action of the notorious nerve gases follows similar lines. Bacteria, too, can attack the synapses. Tetanus toxin, the poison of the tetanus bacilli, blocks inhibiting synapses, so that the muscles lose their capacity for properly co-ordinated movements, and instead develop a compulsive stiffness.

Synapses, however, offer vantage points not only for fatal disturbance from outside but also for desired chemical stimuli. Drugs with which mentally sick patients are treated today, develop their action at synapses, and this is also the case with other psychoactive drugs. In 1970, when the Nobel Prize Committee awarded the prize for medicine to Ulf von Euler, Julius Axelrod and Sir Bernard Katz, the citation said: 'Their discoveries have given an extraordinary impetus to the search for drugs to fight nerve diseases and mental disorders.'

14

The Chemistry of Psychology

'Opium induces sleep,' says a character in Molière's *Le Malade Imaginaire*, 'because it has sleep-power in it.' Such was the simple explanation three hundred years ago for the effect of a psychoactive drug; and even today the layman may feel this is as good a reason as he needs. But for the 'sleep-power' to become effective, of course, it must have a material basis and specific sites of action. The former was established earlier: the effect of a substance on the brain is connected with its chemical structure. But research scientists have only in very recent years been able to achieve well-grounded ideas about the sites of action. Chemical influences from outside depend on the synapses, the junctions at the many points of connection between nerve cells. Here, over a distance of the hundred thousandth of a millimetre, the electrical signal is transformed into a chemical one. In the tiny synaptic gap, or rather in the majority of synaptic gaps, psychoactive drugs can make their influence effective.

Deficiency depression

The action mechanism of anti-depressive drugs has been

particularly well investigated; and it has been shown that they counteract a deficiency in transmitter substances from which depressives suffer.

Investigations on the brains of depressive patients after their death proved that in parts of the brain stem, the diencephalon and the inner cerebral regions, the content of the transmitters noradrenalin and serotonin was greatly reduced during depressions. These and other findings, concerned especially with the metabolism of the two transmitters, with their origin and their structure in the organism, led to development of the idea that a deficiency of them in the appropriate synaptic gaps caused depressions. If there is such a deficiency at crucial places in the brain, the flow of signals is inhibited. It appears fairly certain today that there are close connections between such disorders and the psychological and physical symptoms of the depressions.

One might think that noradrenalin and serotonin could simply be injected somehow into the patients who have a deficiency in these substances; but unfortunately this does not work. For a substance to take effect in the brain, it has to get there; and although these two substances flow to the brain with the bloodstream, they cannot there leave the blood vessels. A mechanism which scientists call 'blood-brain-barrier' stops substances from the blood vessels penetrating indiscriminately into the brain tissue. Even when the brain has a deficiency in noradrenalin and serotonin, they are barred entrance to it.

The brain itself produces its own transmitter substances. Noradrenalin is formed from the amino acid, tyrosine; serotonin from another amino acid, tryptophan. Both amino acids are components of the protein we absorb with our food, and they pass the blood-brain-barrier without any trouble. But tyrosine and tryptophan also failed as anti-depressives. Tyrosine did not help depressive patients at all. With tryptophan doctors achieved some improvements, but not impressive enough to be added to the psychiatrists' pharmacopoeia. Evidently a deficit in the raw materials from which the transmitter substances are formed is not the decisive factor causing a depression.

Anti-depressive drugs, then, do not simply lead to an increase in the transmitter substances. The basic cause of depression seems to be that transmitter substances disappear from the synaptic gap too quickly for use in the orderly transmission of signals. This process is prevented by the anti-depressives.

In normal brain activity the transmitters poured out into the synaptic gap for the transmission of signals are removed again from the gap in two ways. One of them is that an enzyme called monoaminoxydase (MAO for short) turns the transmitter into a substance no longer adapted for signal-carrying. The other way of making the transmitters inactive, which plays a bigger part with noradrenalin and probably with serotonin too, is that they return to the synaptic terminal boutons from which they came.

Anti-depressives intervene at both these points. A group of drugs inhibits the MAO, and consequently, even if Chinese communists might suspect counter-revolutionary activities, they are called MAO-inhibitors. A second group, today the more important therapeutically, acts as a brake on the return of the transmitters into the nerve cell. With this group of drugs the molecular nucleus consists of three mutually connected rings of atoms; so they are called 'tricyclic antidepressives'.

The action of a third group cannot be put into either of these categories. It consists of very simple compounds of the chemical element lithium which, like potassium and sodium, is one of the alkaline metals. As these two elements have a decisive function in transmitting an electric signal into the nerve fibre, it is not surprising that lithium, being closely related, can also influence the cell membrane's activity. So far, however, there is no clear idea of the connections between such effects of lithium and its favourable action on depressive patients.

There are indeed many other questions still unanswered as to the action of the anti-depressives.

'Why', asks Norbert Matussek of the Max Planck Institute for Psychiatry in Munich, 'does it take from eight to eighteen days before the anti-depressive effect on the patient is visible? . . . Why do only some of the depressive patients respond to the various drugs? Do the patients have other metabolism disorders which are not cured by the drugs used today? . . . How are these processes affected by acetylcholine (another important transmitter substance)?'

Still, it has basically been proved—and this is a crucial principle—that specific disorders in the brain's metabolism, that is chemical processes, are connected with the agonising psychological symptoms of depression. That scientists working in this field have not yet discovered all the exact details is no wonder considering one great limitation on their work. They cannot do the most obvious thing for a researcher. As Matussek says: 'It would be extremely enlightening to analyse various brain areas of particular interest for the depression; but on ethical and legal grounds it is impossible on living depressive patients to obtain brain matter from specially important regions.'

In view of this limitation, which of course applies also to investigations on the effect of other psychoactive drugs, researchers are left mainly with two unsatisfactory possibilities: chemical studies on the brains of dead patients and investigating the live brains of animals. But dead brains no longer show the metabolism concerned, and the 'psychology' of animals is very different from that of man; where there are common factors, it is hard to take them into account because animals can't talk about their experiences! So discoveries have to be made piecemeal by roundabout ways. Put together, they so far show only the broad outlines of the picture; that is already something.

Differences of effect

There are other psychoactive drugs which ensure that there is more noradrenalin in the synaptic gap. The amphetamines release noradrenalin from the storage vesicle and at the same time block its return into the vesicle. Some of the stimulating effect of cocaine is also based on the forcing of noradrenalin out of the nerve cell and the inhibiting of its return. The action of caffein, too, is caused by the release of transmitter substance.

Between a cup of coffee and a sniff of cocaine, an amphetamine and an anti-depressant, there are considerable differences of effect. But considering that all four are stimulating drugs, it is less surprising that they lead to a similar result, an increase of noradrenalin in the synaptic gap. The differences of effect may arise from the fact that the intervention on the noradrenalin metabolism occurs at different places. Psychoactive drugs may influence the composition of the substance, its release from the storage vesicle, the activity of MAO and of another component enzyme, or its return to the vesicle. It is also important, no doubt, how intense an influence a drug has on the noradrenalin metabolism. But even more important are the other effects it may have on the brain: on the serotonin metabolism, or a number of other transmitter substances about whose function very little is known.

An excess of effective transmitter substance leads to states of excitement. Although there is still controversy about the causes of schizophrenia, whose victims suffer from severe agitation, delusions and hallucinations, it has been proved that the analeptics, with which schizophrenics nowadays can be effectively helped, suppress the activity of the transmitter substances. One of these drugs, reserpine, can even lead to a condition which looks very like a depression. On the other hand, continual abuse of the stimulant amphetamines may cause clinical conditions similar to schizophrenia with severe agitation and mental confusion.

Chemical causes of hallucinations?

In view of the uncertainty on details which prevails today, there is little point in discussing here what chemical action in the brain is known or presumed for the other psychoactive drugs. But it is worth mentioning a few interesting common features.

A whole number of hallucinogens show a similar chemical structure to serotonin. They include the active substances in the Mexican 'holy mushroom' and LSD. Mescalin, the active substance in the peyote cactus, is closely related chemically to noradrenalin. The muscarinic agent contained in fly agaric is like the transmitter substance acetylcholine in its molecular structure.

The similarity of molecular structure in hallucinogens and transmitter substances can scarcely be a coincidence. But what do we deduce from that? According to an interesting speculation, the hallucinogens work in the brain like transmitter substances and reinforce the amount of real transmitters. As a result the known effect of the hallucinogens occurs: an unusual abundance of feelings, images and ideas appear, which normally are suppressed so that the brain can concentrate on the particular tasks it has to master.

'Among the typical experiences in LSD or mescalin trips,' writes the Munich psychologist Wolfgang Schmidbauer, 'one is that consciousness is flooded with incredibly intense perceptions and all the senses communicate far richer and more plentiful messages than is biologically expedient. The LSD or mescalin "tripper" is in fact less efficient biologically, because he is impressed and carried away by a wealth of unwanted experiences. We may conclude from this that we are normally aware of only a small but appropriate and constant section of all our sense impressions.'

But not all hallucinogens are chemically related to the transmitter substances so far known; and most of the substances which show a similar structure to the transmitters do not cause any hallucinations. This alone gives an impression of the range of problems still to be solved. It will need still greater efforts before the most important connections in the chemistry of the brain are fully understood.

On the fundamental importance of chemical processes for our psychology, however, there is no longer any doubt, however much it goes against the grain of our ideas. 'Nature', remarks Schmidbauer, 'passes indifferently over a central feature of our conceptions about ourselves and our environment. It ignores the fact that we experience psychological processes as something quite different from material phenomena.'

15

Secret Order in the Jungle

To recapitulate some of the facts discovered by brain researchers: For the achievements of our brain, both those we take for granted and those of which we are specially proud as human beings, the thousand million nerve cells in our head are responsible. They are the basic elements in brain activity. But each nerve cell is also a small universe in itself: a highly organised system showing characteristic features besides those typical of all living cells.

Every nerve cell possesses several branching dendrites and one nerve fibre with thin branches, at some distance from the cell body, each ending as the terminal bouton of a synapse. All nerve cells receive electric signals, transmit them to the nerve fibre and along it to the terminal boutons, which with the aid of chemical conversion processes see it is passed on to the adjoining cells. And since both exciting and inhibiting signals are continually arriving, a nerve cell finds out at every moment whether a signal is to be transmitted or not. It acts as a calculating machine, which is permanently adding and subtracting electric potentials.

Assuming we know everything about the nerve cell's structure and function (which of course we certainly do not despite the amazing discoveries which scientists have already made), and assuming all the chemical processes in the brain were familiar to us down to the smallest details (and that is even further from the case), would all the riddles of the brain be solved?

Not at all. We should still be missing a crucial condition for understanding the human brain: the 'wiring diagram'. The ten thousand million or more nerve cells crammed closely together to form our brain cannot be connected at random. The nerve cell jungle revealed by the microscopic preparations must have a secret order, however arbitrary the connections appear to be. D. Whitteridge of Edinburgh University has expressed the opinion of many brain researchers: 'We would undoubtedly understand by now how the brain works, if we had a wiring diagram which showed the connections of its ten thousand million cells, and if we knew which ones were exciting, which inhibiting.'

But if such a diagram were there, it would be hard enough for experts to find their way through it.

'We would of course group many nerve fibres together, much as one might group together all the trunk lines running from Manchester to London, and say that all these pathways have much the same function, only differing in the exchange from which they originated. In this way, the nerve fibres running from the eye to the brain have much the same function, but some arise from the centre of the retina and others from the periphery. Even with this simplification, however, we should still find the wiring diagram too vast for comprehension, and we should have to break it up, as electronic engineers do, into block diagrams which describe the function and the interconnections of each part, without worrying about the wiring inside each block.'

Some figures will show the difficulties faced by researchers who try to unravel the wiring diagram of the human brain. If every one of the ten thousand million nerve cells is connected with only a thousand others (up to 100,000 synapses have been estimated for a single nerve cell), that makes ten billion (million million) connections, a figure at which most people's minds will boggle. I will try to make it more concrete.

Let us assume that the human brain's wiring diagram is known and a working party has the task of constructing a magnified model of the brain connections with ten billion contact points—say as an advertisement for a world exhibition. Standardised building parts have to be prefabricated, the delivery smoothly organised. One group of workers must be exclusively concerned with inserting in the model the contact points corresponding to the synapses in the brain. Each of these workers has to install a contact point without a break every ten seconds, during a forty-two-hour week. (We can safely reckon with a forty-two-hour week, because with this working period in a seven-day week four men share a work-place; for convenience I leave out of account holidays and sickness.) Question: How many workers will be needed round the clock in shift-work if the model with the ten billion contact points is to be completed in ten years' continuous work? Answer: about 1,300,000.

Such a model would not be built even then if the human brain's wiring diagram were successfully discovered without gaps. Brain researchers freely admit that they are still a very long way from such a stage of knowledge. Measured by the size of the task, in fact, only the first steps have so far been taken. But what has already come out of these deserves attention, not least because such investigations have made it clear how very much the brain's activity depends on the right connections between the nerve cells.

Reflexes and conditioned reflexes

Basic discoveries about the simplest connections have been made in parts of the nervous system outside the brain.

There is, for instance, the well-known knee-joint reflex to examine the patient for certain nerve complaints. The doctor taps with a small hammer on the soft place under the knee-cap, and the lower leg shoots upwards in an involuntary movement. Such a movement taking place automatically, a reflex in fact, is made possible by a connection which is called a reflex arc.

What happens at the testing of the knee-joint reflex? The tap from the hammer hits a joint connecting the extensor muscle in the thigh with the shinbone. Through the blow on the joint the extensor muscle becomes a little stretched. The stretching causes a nerve signal which is transmitted to the spinal cord. It is there processed with the aim of balancing the effect of the hammer blow. On a second nerve path a signal travels back to the extensor muscle giving the instruction: contract again at once. This happens, and as a result the lower leg shoots upwards.

Reflexes are reactions of the body which are not improved by reflection. On the contrary, it is often the case that something happens at once without any hesitation. If we accidentally touch a hot-plate with the hand, fractions of a second may be decisive for the extent of the burn. Many warning signals causing reflex movements are therefore not processed first in the brain but already in the spinal cord. The movements take place blindly, but then the brain clarifies the situation.

It is promptly informed of the occurrence, and, then, after the reflex movement, has to find out in more detail what has happened and decide whether further actions are necessary. The knee-joint reflex might be produced not by the tap of the doctor's hammer but by some different cause. A defence reaction might be indicated, more care in making other movements, or flight.

We live with a mass of reflexes. A grain of dust flies into the eye: we at once begin to blink, and tear fluid is secreted to wash away the dust. We step out of a dark room into the light: the pupils contract. Some food gets into the windpipe: the cough reflex engages. The rectum fills: the sphincter contracts. There are swallowing and choking reflexes, reflexes to control breathing and circulation, stomach and bowel movements, to discharge saliva, bile, stomach juices. Over twenty thousand reflex paths, it is estimated, protect the organism and ensure as smooth as possible a course for the processes of life, without the brain being continually called on for decisions.

Not all reflex curves represent such simple connections as the one for which the knee-joint reflex is responsible. A complex control mechanism regulates the width of the pupils. The brightness of the light falling on the light-sensitive cells of the retina is registered, and an average brightness is worked out, which as an electrical signal travels down certain nerve fibres to enter a region in the brain stem. There a balance takes place between what the brightness is and what it 'ought to be'. By a second nerve path a signal goes to the eye which—according to the conditions of the light—produces a contraction or expansion of the pupil.

This control, which is continually being exercised, is like the mechanism with which the activity of a central heating system is controlled. A thermostat automatically switches on the heating when the temperature sinks below a certain point, and switches if off again when the temperature rises above that point. The pupil reflex functions, in fact, like many other regulation processes in the body (including regulation of body temperature). It works on the same principle as many other technical devices besides central heating systems which are automatically adapted to chang-ing demands. Brain researchers as well as engineers talk of 'negative feedback'.

Many reflexes include whole programmes. When we are startled by an unexpected loud noise, the 'surprise reflex' occurs. We feel as if we are merely giving a start, but in reality the reaction is far more differentiated: we pull in the head and close the eyes, bring the elbows into the body and bend the knees a bit. If the shock is great enough, the blood pressure rises, and changes in the metabolism mobilise energy for fight or flight. Such a reflex, which has its effect in many parts of the body, presupposes complex connections which are not yet known.

All the reflexes so far known are innate, but they can also be acquired, as was shown by the famous experiments of the Russian physiologist Ivan Pavlov at the beginning of this century. In St. Petersburg Pavlov investigated in dogs first the processes which take place in digestion—work for which in 1904 he was awarded the Nobel Prize. He based his experiments on the fact that saliva glands are activated by food, as human mouths 'water' when food is put on the table.

Pavlov's main distinction as a brain researcher lies in the discovery that it does not need the food to set in motion the secretion of saliva. For some time he made a bell ring just before the dogs were fed, till eventually the sound was enough to produce the flow of saliva. The reflex had occurred at a signal which was not originally envisaged as a stimulator in the brain's connections. Pavlov called it a 'conditioned reflex'.

Further investigations showed that all kinds of different stimulators can be coupled with all kinds of reflexes, in men as well. In an experiment reported by C. V. Hudgins, very bright light was beamed into the test subject's eyes, causing the pupil reflex: the pupils contracted. Directly before the light was switched on, a bell rang. After this procedure had been repeated several times, the sound of the bell was enough to produce a contraction of the pupils.

Hudgins then went a step further. Whenever the bell rang, he said loudly: 'contract'. Eventually he could do without the bell; the reflex seemed to occur on command. Yet the subject was unaware of any deliberate action. When asked by Hudgins 'What did you do when I said "contract"?', the regular answer was: 'I didn't do anything.'

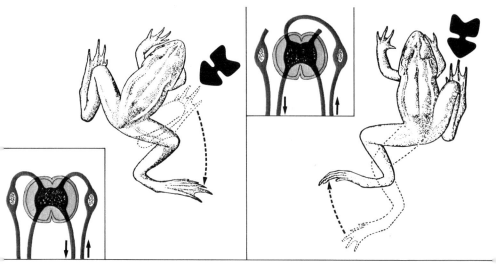

A frog which has its right rear leg tickled withdraws this leg. The afferent sensation nerve from the right rear leg transmits the stimulus to a centre in the spinal cord, which causes the leg movement by way of the afferent motor nerve. The pictures left show the normal connection and the frog's reaction. With the frog (right) the afferent nerve of the right rear leg was connected to the nerve centre which normally processes the sensations from the left rear leg. The wrong connection makes the frog withdraw the left leg when tickled on the right leg.

The conditioned reflex, too, must be the result of a definite connection; for it to function promptly the conditioning must first be achieved by a learning process. It has not been discovered whether completely new connections between nerve cells are produced or whether it involves connections there from the beginning. Some researchers who thought they had found in the conditioned reflex the key for the whole complex of brain activity were certainly over-hasty in their conclusions.

Interference with the connections

It has been repeatedly shown in experiments how very much even the simplest reflexes are dependent on the right connections. Before Roger Sperry and his colleagues in Los Angeles started splitting brains, he was working on the wiring plans of the nervous system. He deliberately disturbed the connections (along lines previously tested) so as to observe the consequences. He distorted the normal brain circuitry so that the wrong nerve cells became connected.

With frogs, for instance, he severed the two nerves which transmit sensations from the rear legs to the spinal cord, and then connected the sensation of the right rear leg to the centre in the spinal cord which normally processes the sensations from the left rear leg. The frogs, which before the operation had withdrawn the right leg when tickled there, now reacted to the stimulus in the right leg by withdrawing the left one. The signal 'it's tickling' had simply gone to the wrong place.

Sperry produced these wrong connections in rats by a similar operation adapted to the different anatomical conditions. Like the frogs, the rats reacted with the left leg when it should have been the right. They were standing on a wire grid, and he stimulated their right rear leg with a slight shock from below. The left leg at once jerked upwards. Some rats had a sore place on the sole of their right rear paw. They limped through the cage on three legs, but it was the unaffected left leg they tried to spare by lifting it. They also licked this leg, obviously feeling pain; and paid no attention to the right leg with its bad paw.

Although such experiments have never been tried on men, there is no doubt that the same kind of wrong connection would make us jerk the left leg instead of the right. Similar macabre effects have in fact been observed with patients who suffered from the consequences of wrong connections after nerve injuries through accidents.

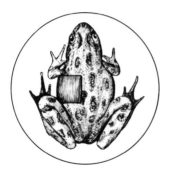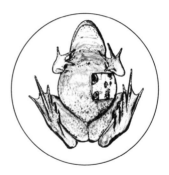

*If a strip of skin is cut out of a tadpole and transplanted, it heals up
there, even if the belly end is now on the back, the back end on the belly.
Tests with the grown frog show that the nerve connections to the piece of
skin removed and reinserted have been restored again exactly as before
the operation.*

In man and the higher animals severed nerve fibres do not
grow together again; but only a few hours after the injury
regeneration processes start at the stump of the fibre which
is still connected with the cell body. The fibres begin to grow
at a speed of from half to four millimetres a day and gradually
penetrate into an area temporarily cut off from nerve connections. Sometimes, however, the nerve fibres sprout in
the wrong direction. There are reports, for instance, of
patients in whom the newly-grown nerve fibres reached the
tear glands instead of the appropriate saliva glands; when
food was put on the table and saliva production should have
been caused, the patients couldn't help crying. In other
cases branches of tongue or shoulder nerves grew into face
parts, resulting in grotesque twitches of the face which
occurred after movements of the tongue or the shoulder
muscles.

Luckily the right connections are restored as a rule. In
lower vertebrates this happens with amazing completeness.
Sperry's former colleague Nancy Miner cut out a strip of
tadpoles' skin from a place on the body reaching from the

middle of the belly to the middle of the back, and transplanted it so that the end of the belly was now on the back
and the end of the back on the belly. When the tadpoles
had turned into frogs, they reacted very strikingly. If they
were tickled on the part of the back where the piece of skin
had been removed and transplanted to right the other side
of the body, they scratched their belly with one leg. Touching
the belly, on the other hand, made them scratch their back.

So the severed nerve connections to the transplanted
piece of skin must have been restored exactly as they were
before the operation. The sensation nerves on the belly must
have grown to the belly end of the strip of skin which was
now at the back. A touch there produced the nerve signal
'touch on the belly' and caused the appropriate scratching
movement.

Even more astonishing are the results of experiments in
which Sperry severed frogs' optic nerves and at the same
time turned the eyes in their sockets round 180°. After a
while the frogs could see again; only now the world stood
on its head for them, without the brain being aware of this.
If a fly buzzed above them, they did not jump for it, but
lowered their head to snap at it.

Incredible as it may sound, at the regeneration of the
connections between the eyes and the appropriate parts of
the brain, thousands or even millions of nerve fibres, which
are converted into electrical signals and transmit visual
impressions into the brain, must have been exactly recon-
nected with their original destination; only the position of
the eye after its reversal was no longer correct. Because of
this the retina was falsely lighted, and the brain, despite—
or rather just because of—being rightly connected again
with the retina, could not cause behaviour adapted to the
real situation.

Sperry then went a step further. With his colleague
Domenica Attardi he severed the optic nerves of goldfish
and at the same time removed a part of the light-sensitive

retina from which many nerve fibres entered the optic nerve leading to the brain. They thereby deprived the individual fish of different parts of their retina. After three weeks, when the connections to the brain were restored and the goldfish could see again, Sperry and his colleague killed them and examined their brains. A special colouring process made it possible to recognise clearly the freshly-grown nerve fibres. Since the fish had been left with different parts of the retina, the experiments could follow up which parts were newly connected with which regions of the brain. And it proved that the nerve fibres had infallibly grown towards the regions designed in each case. Sperry commented: 'It is as if the forces of the embryonic development which arranged the connections in the beginning continue to be effective at the regeneration.'

Unfortunately a man whose optic nerve has been broken off by an accident cannot expect that he will one day see again. We have lost the capacity for renewing parts of the body (as an earthworm or starfish can), and the regeneration capacity of our nerve connections is also limited. Yet other observations by brain researchers leave no doubt that, with man as well, every point in the retina is connected with a specific point in the cerebrum.

Research on snails

In view of the immense number of nerve cells and their connections in the human brain, researchers wishing to study the connections have looked round for better subjects. Mammal brains were little more use, and even the relatively primitive brains of frogs and fishes have far too complex a structure for connection researchers. So they climbed further down the evolutionary tree till they came to organisms with simply organised nervous systems which seemed to offer better prospects for the attempt at exact analysis.

They began to investigate the nerve nodes of leeches, crabs, insects and, above all, large sea-snails. The nerve cells of those creatures do not amount to thousands of millions, as with man, but 'only' to thousands. The snails also looked attractive as subjects for research, because their nerve cells are relatively huge: the diameter is up to a millimetre.

The American zoologist A. O. D. Willows, for instance, is studying the nervous system of a large sea-snail called triton (Latin name *Tritonia*) which is over thirty centimetres long. He set out to become familiar with the connections whereby Tritonia can escape from a hungry starfish in a flight reaction lasting about thirty seconds and activating large parts of the body. He was able to identify dozens of separate nerve cells by their characteristic size or colour in the brain, and to recognise them repeatedly.

After identifying a good number of cells and giving them code names, he stimulated with electric current over thirty neuronal axons, and through a very fine electrode monitored the identified cells to find out whether the artificial signal arrived. This produced over twenty thousand measurements; and the same number resulted from reversing the procedure: he stimulated the nerve cells and monitored the fibre cords. Finally he investigated whether signals could be exchanged between two identified nerve cells. Despite this massive operation, Willows cannot yet present a complete wiring plan for Tritonia's flight reaction. He is optimistic, however, that this project, followed by others building on the results, will in due course be successful. He wrote in 1971:

'There is reason to be confident that within a few years the cellular exploration of the nervous systems of Tritonia and other simple animals will provide a clear enough under-standing of their nervous apparatus and mechanisms to describe these systems in the definitive terms usually reserved for man-made machines. These investigations should also help greatly in determining the general relations between the brain and behaviour in the vast number of simple animal species comprising most of the animal kingdom—and ultimately in more complex animals.'

Although man too may be called a more complicated species of animal, Willows was no doubt thinking of fishes and frogs. It appears very unlikely today that the connections of the human brain will be unravelled within a foreseeable period, even though all the experts agree on their great importance for understanding the activity of that brain.

Psychiatrists have learnt to value the chemical aspects of their discipline, since psychoactive drugs made them feel far better equipped to help their patients; but they must take into account that a mental illness may also be the result of wrong connections in the brain. Seymour Kety of Massachussetts General Hospital, Boston, talking of the search for the causes of schizophrenia, said the possibility should not be ignored that 'hereditary factors in schizophrenics have led to inappropriate connection paths or action variations between chemically normal parts of the brain. Should this be the case, the physiological psychologist, neurophysiologist or anatomist will probably make important discoveries long before the biochemist. Many biochemists would take a long time to find a short-circuit in a radio receiver if they were confined to chemical techniques.'

Not all brain researchers go as far as Roger Sperry, who declares that 'the essential secrets of learning and memory, as of the higher brain functions altogether, are situated on the level of the brain connections'; he is unimpressed by the knowledge gained about the activity of individual nerve cells. This knowledge for him means no more than 'the knowledge of the chemical components of the printer's ink and paper which have been used to print a message in an unknown language'.

Gene manipulation

If difficult connections play as large a part in the brain as experts think, an extremely high proportion of our genes must be alone responsible for the development and maintenance of the correct connections between the nerve cells. These genes, which are contained in the germ cells of father and mother and which join up on fertilisation to form the structural plan for the newly emerging life, decide that a human being and not, say, a fly, an elephant or any other creature develops out of the fertilised egg cell. They also provide the blue-print of the individual characteristics which distinguish each person from his fellow humans. What this means for the brain is that heredity must be responsible at least in part both for the connections which every human brain possesses and also for those which decide talent, temperament and other mental and psychological qualities of the individual.

The hypothesis that a considerable part of our genes are concerned with the brain was confirmed in 1971 by two American researchers, William Han and Charles Laird respectively of Colorado and Texas universities. In complex biochemical investigations they tested the genetic make-up of mice. This showed that at least three hundred thousand genes, about a tenth of the mouse's whole inheritance, relate to the brain, as against only three per cent for other organs such as liver and kidneys, with just as difficult and complex tasks. Since man and mouse differ above all in the organisation of their brains, it may be expected that with man a far larger proportion of the inheritance is devoted to the brain.

Gene manipulation, the long-discussed futurologist's dream of deliberately modifying hereditary qualities, would certainly give extensive possibilities—once that stage is reached—for influencing the development of brains. But important preconditions for teaching it are still missing. Geneticists do not know enough about the position of the genes on the chromosomes, nor have they methods to allow such manipulation. Moreover, since so little is known about the brain's connections, and even less about the relations between connections and functions, there is a complete lack of definite aims for changes in the genes which affect the brain.

Discoveries in glass dishes

To get nearer the secret of the brain connections, scientists, especially in the United States, have started to breed what *Time* magazine called 'Brain in the Test Tube'. Admittedly the word 'Brain' is a great exaggeration at this stage in the experiments, and the glass containers used by the researchers are not test tubes. But the results achieved, especially by experiments in the National Institutes of Health at Bethesda near Washington, are exciting enough. They allowed basic processes taking place in the brain and in other parts of the nervous system to be observed in cell cultures.

One of the researchers at Bethesda, Gerald Fischbach, removed parts of the tissue of chicken embryos from the spinal cord, and he then separated the nerve cells through a technique tested by other researchers. As a result of a special chemical treatment the still embryonic cells, which did not yet show the typical ramifications of mature nerve cells, lost their connection to each other, without suffering any injury. The separate cells thus gained were distributed by Fischbach into shallow glass Petri dishes in which the cells were given all the food substances necessary.

From the nerve cells nerve fibres were soon sprouting, which sought contact with other nerve cells. Groups of nerve cells formed connections with each other. At the contact points Fischbach proved that there were synapses, and through them electric potentials were transmitted:

information in the language which only nerve cells understand. The nerve cells released by the researchers from the society of nerves had created a community of signals in the glass dish. In effect, then, the British journal *New Scientist* declared enthusiastically, 'Fischbach has . . . succeeded in recreating the vital wiring and connections that enable us to move and think, and all this in Petri dishes on his laboratory bench.'

In another experiment Fischbach provided company for the isolated nerve cells in the form of isolated muscle cells of chicken embryos. While the nerve cells developed nerve fibres, the muscle cells grew up to normal striate muscle fibres. Would the nerve fibres, as is the case in the body, come into connection with the muscle fibres and make them suddenly contract through electric signals? Yes, nerve cells in the glass dish produced violent contractions of muscle fibres.

That isolated nerve cells outside the body evidently connect with each other is no peculiarity of nerve cells from chicken embryos. In other laboratories the nerve cells of mice embryos also did what was expected of them. Richard Sidman at Harvard removed the nerve cells from the embryonic brains of 'reeler' mice, which through a serious hereditary defect reel as if drunk when they run: this is caused by wrong connections in the cerebellum and the cerebral cortex. The artificially separated cells of these brains with their hereditary defect also joined up again in the glass bowls, but in a different connection pattern from that formed by the nerve cells of normal mice—in the 'reeler' pattern. Are there perhaps conditions under which nerve cells of reeler mice produce normal connections to each other? Questions like these can be investigated on the brain tissue cultivated in Petri dishes.

The possibility of exposing brain tissue to various chemical and physical influences, and under conditions where the changes can be well observed, will clearly enjoy great popularity among brain researchers. Such brain studies in Petri dishes offer prospects of important new discoveries about the human brain as well—and certainly increase, too, the range of possibilities for brain manipulation.

16

The Brain as Data-Processor

Brain researchers no longer compare the brain's functioning with that of a telephone exchange, for there is clearly a fundamental difference: in a telephone system the importance of a message transmitted depends on the transmitter, in the brain on the receiver.

'When I pick out a telephone number and give a message,' says the British brain researcher W. Grey Walter, 'the message remains the same even if I give it to the wrong number. The result of such a mistake in the brain, however, is quite different. . . . Let us assume that some vinegar comes into contact with a taste-bud on the tongue and picks up a "wrong lead"—for instance, the nerve fibre which passes on the stimulus produced by vinegar is not connected with its proper receiving area but somehow cut off and plugged in to a nerve fibre leading from the ear to the brain—what would one then taste? One would hear a very loud and frightening noise. Every time the nerve ending in the tongue was stimulated, one would have the same hallucination. If, instead, an acoustic nerve were wrongly connected with an optic nerve, one would have visual sensations instead of hearing music.'

What flows into the brain from the sense organs is not images or sounds, tastes or smells, but only electrical signals. The signals are coded messages, but how the messages are interpreted depends on the receiving place. Thus the visual centre understands only 'light', while for the hearing centre every signal means a noise. Because that is the case, Robert White (as described in Chapter 1) could make the monkey's brain peeled from its skull 'see' and 'hear' something, although he had deprived it of its eyes and ears: he merely transmitted some current into the stumps of optic and acoustic nerves.

Brain and computer

Is the brain anything like a computer? At first sight there is much to be said for this analogy. The computer, like the brain, is fed information in coded form; both process the information and pass it on. Computer technicians speak of input and output and of data processing for what happens in between. These expressions can also be used for the activity of the brain. Moreover, both computer and brain have a store of information, which is essential to them for data processing, which in turn cannot be satisfactorily carried out without the right, highly complicated connections.

But there are notable differences, too, between a computer and a brain. Materially, the chief components of a computer are made of metal, while the brain is composed of living cells. The brain is tiny compared with a computer, but has

These nerve cells are to be found in the outer layers of the brain—in the cerebral cortex. They are much more closely packed there than in this schematised illustration, and their countless, finely branched dendrites are as interwoven as the undergrowth of adjoining bushes. The nerve cells are in contact solely through the piston-shaped structures, the synapses.

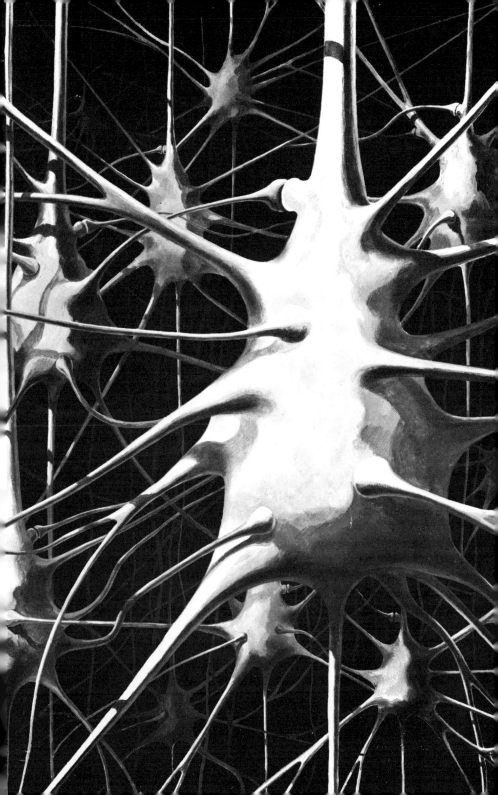

an incomparably greater 'performance'. In its powers, the computer beats a human brain for mastering specific problems which can be automatically solved. It is better at calculation—appropriately programmed, of course, by brains. Its memory works infallibly. The brain, on the other hand, is infinitely more versatile, and its activity produces not only solid output, but phenomena which no computers offer at present and which they are very unlikely to offer in the future, however efficient: emotions, creative thinking, will-power, consciousness.

So despite the similarities, it seems wise not to press the computer analogy very far. It is understandable that a scientist like Sir John Eccles, who has made it his life's work to investigate the interaction of nerve cells, should take a critical view of the analogy:

'I would like to state that no insight into the mode of working of the nervous system can be gained if one starts from the premise that it functions like a metal computer. This analogy with the computer rests on a superficial similarity with the process of input and output and may be disastrously misleading.'

Harmony through the cerebellum

The computer image really fits best for a part of the brain which has attracted less attention through spectacular experiments than brain stem, diencephalon and cerebrum: the cerebellum. We know most about the circuitry of the cerebellum—it is the only part, in fact, for which scientists have been able to discover the connections to any degree worth mentioning. We owe this knowledge above all to Eccles and his colleagues; but even they would have made little progress if the cerebellum had not had a relatively simple structure, with the same pattern of nerve cells repeated over and over again. 'In it', says Eccles, 'there is a wonderfully geometrical arrangement of unique nerve elements.'

Sticking out from the brain stem into the back of the head, covered by the cerebrum, the cerebellum weighs 120 grams (a little over 4 oz.,) about ten times less than the cerebrum. Like the cerebrum, it consists of grey and white matter. The thin cortical layer containing the nerve cells is grey; the interior, made up of nerve fibres, is white.

The surface of the cerebellum is furrowed like the cerebrum, but the furrows go far deeper. They even have thin branches. This aesthetic nature of its structure made some anatomists of the Middle Ages think it was the seat of the soul. Modern researchers find it remarkable that, because of the deep furrowing, the surface occupied by the grey cortex in the cerebellum, though so much smaller than the cerebrum, is far more extended proportionately, about 1000 square centimetres as against 2500 for the surface of the cerebrum.

The importance of the cerebellum was conclusively proved decades ago through the results of animal experiments in which parts of it were removed, and through observations on human patients with a cerebellum damaged by injuries or tumours. Both animals and men reveal damage to the cerebellum by striking motor disorders. They reel about as if drunk, their movements are jerky and unco-ordinated, overshoot their aim and are completely lacking in suppleness, let alone elegance. A normal person can easily find the tip of his nose with his forefinger when his eyes are closed. A patient with a damaged cerebellum brings his finger near to the nose with quivering movements which become more and more violent, and will sometimes bang his hand into his face.

The cerebellum has the function of co-ordinating all movements for harmonious execution—a function far less trivial than our everyday experience would at first suggest to us. Merely to clench the fist needs the interaction of

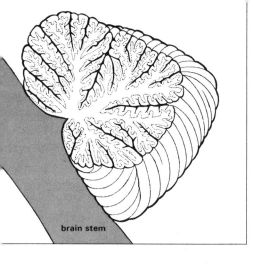

The cerebellum (shown here in sections) is deeply furrowed. Because of this it has a very large surface, which—as with the cerebrum—is made up of grey cortex.

brain stem

a whole number of muscles which must contract or expand at the right moment and with the right strength. When we run or jump, most of the five hundred-odd skeletal muscles in our body come into action. By directives precisely attuned to each other, the cerebellum ensures that the movements of the individual muscles complement each other satisfactorily.

As explained in Chapter 5, a strip of cerebral cortex, known as motor cortex, is very important for movements. But the cerebrum evidently has to bother itself only while movements and movement processes are new and have to be learnt. Everyone knows how strenuous it is to learn swimming, dancing, cycling or skating. The beginner is obliged to attend to all his bodily movements, which are usually carried out automatically and do not require any sort of attention. The unwonted movements are at first uncertain and stiff. Only by constant concentration does he gradually succeed in making the many muscles involved work together harmoniously.

The cerebrum now tries to dispose as soon as possible of the task which demands so much concentration from it. It hands the task over to the cerebellum, gaining freedom for more interesting activity: for instance, watching the road while cycling, day-dreaming while skating, or flirting while dancing! Only the general guide-lines for a deliberate movement are still given by the cerebrum. The cerebellum works out the precise plan and supervises the course of the movements. It is therefore connected with the motor cortex, the muscles and the sense organs of the skin, but also with the organ of balance, the eyes, the ears, and the centres in the cerebrum responsible for seeing and hearing. All these connections travel by the path which connects the cerebellum with the brain stem.

On the cerebellar cortex, as on the motor cortex of the cerebrum, there are rules governing the distribution of 'responsibilities'. Brain researchers have been able, in fact, to make out three cortical half-men on the cerebellar cortex: one has the shape of somebody lying flat with all his limbs spread-eagled, the other two are like sitting figures linked together at the back like Siamese twins.

The circuit of the cerebellum

Because of its structure, repeated in a relatively uniform way, which can be recognised under the microscope, the cerebellum offered the most favourable starting-point for learning details of the wiring diagram. The results of laborious investigations revealed well-ordered conditions, but they too were discouragingly complicated.

The grey cerebellar cortex consists everywhere of three layers. Between the 'molecular layer' outside and the 'granular layer' inside, there is a simple border layer of nerve cells which are called Purkinje cells after their discoverer. The white matter in the interior of the cerebellum contains nerve fibres, which bring up the input of other parts of the brain, that is the information processed in the cerebral cortex, and which transmit the output, the directives to the muscles and the 'completion reports' to the cerebrum. Input enters the cerebellum by two sorts of nerve fibres, which are called 'mossy fibres' and 'climbing fibres'. Output leaves the cerebellum by only one way: through the nerve fibres of the thick Purkinje cells. What happens to the input in the cerebellar cortex before it becomes output is fantastic.

Each of the branching mossy fibres is connected with hundreds of 'granular cells', a type of nerve cell in the cerebellar cortex which gives the granular layer its name. Branches of different mossy fibres come together also in the same granular cell.

Like all nerve cells, the granular cells are equipped with several dendrites and one nerve fibre, and like all nerve cells they receive electrical signals with the dendrites and transmit them through the nerve fibres and over synapses to other nerve cells. The nerve fibre of each granular cell thrusts straight outwards, between the Purkinje cells and through into the molecular layer. There the nerve fibre splits up and extends to right and left like the crossbeam of a 'T'. This 'crossbeam', called 'parallel fibres', has in its turn many branches, which spread out widely, their tips connected with many other nerve cells to which electrical signals have been passed on.

As message-receivers from the parallel fibres, there are first the dendrites of the Purkinje cells, each of which in the molecular layer forms an extended and thick branch of dendrites, rather like the wall-trees in a summerhouse. The dendrites of each single Purkinje cell connect with the parallel fibres of at least a hundred thousand granular cells; and all transmit signals.

More than that, the parallel fibres excite three more types of nerve cells, basket cells, star cells and Golgi cells (the last, of course, also named after their discoverer), which for their part have an inhibiting effect on adjoining nerve cells. Basket cells and star cells exert their inhibiting influence on Purkinje cells, a whole number of them at a time. Golgi cells, on the other hand, inhibit granular cells, just the type of cell by which they have been excited.

We must now recall that the input reaches the cerebellum

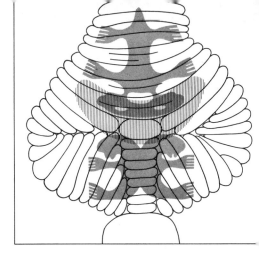

Brain researchers have made out three 'cortical homunculi' in the cerebellar cortex corresponding to the responsibility of the nerve cells for particular bodily regions. In the cross-hatched area acoustic and optical stimuli are received.

by a second way: over the climbing fibres. They are turned diagonally to the Purkinje cells. Usually one climbing fibre at a time accompanies a Purkinje cell, as a creeper climbs a tree. The climbing fibre branches out and follows the dendrites of the Purkinje cell right to the thinnest branches. There are many synapses connecting the climbing fibre with the Purkinje cell, which transmits an incredible drum-fire of signals, both exciting and inhibiting, to create output-directives for muscular movements. Eccles considers the climbing fibres a 'wonderfully arranged system' to test continually the level of excitability of the Purkinje cells, which occupy a central position in the activity of the cerebellum.

When specialists are describing the relations between the various types of nerve cells, the description is full of terms from cybernetics. In what Eccles calls 'a very simplified mode of presentation', for instance, there are sentences like 'The negative feedback via Golgi cells suppresses all feed forward of the granular cells via parallel fibres, not only the excitation of Purkinje cells, but also the negative feedback from the Golgi cells and the negative feed forward from the basket cells and star cells.' This example is only meant to show how far cyberneticist thinking and vocabulary can be used today for processes in the brain. 'It is possible', declared Eccles, 'to describe in schematic form the essential

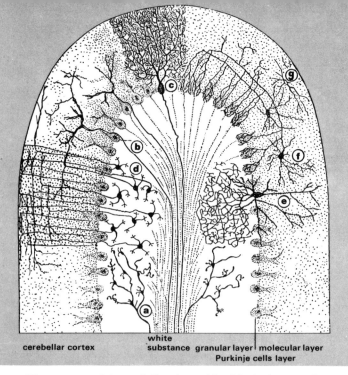

cerebellar cortex

white
substance granular layer | molecular layer
Purkinje cells layer

The structure of the cerebellum is considered by brain researchers
relatively simple and clearly arranged. But it is still discouragingly
complicated, as this schematised drawing of a tiny section of it shows.
Two kinds of nerve fibres, mossy fibres (a) and climbing fibres (b),
transmit the information for processing, the input, to the cerebellum.
The output leaves the cerebellum only by nerve fibres of the bulky
Purkinje cells (c). Involved in the data processing are also granular cells
(d), Golgi cells (e), basket cells (f) and star cells (g).

characteristics of the neuronal circuit (in the cerebellum)'.

Is consciousness, are feeling and thinking, simply the
result of complicated connections between the nerve cells?
No one today can answer this question. There are no other
hypotheses as to where we might look for the secret, especially
the secret of consciousness. If the connections are the
crucial factor, will it one day be possible to build computers
which through their connections possess a consciousness?

Eccles simply excludes such questions from his thought.
He writes: 'Neurophysiology is developed today to a degree

where if in the light of its discoveries we seek any place for a consciousness, we are looking into a void. As neurophysiologists we do not pay any attention at all to consciousness in our conception of the brain's mode of functioning; we go on and on studying these clear neuronal connections, without wondering whether the answers received have anything whatever to do with consciousness.'

This is no doubt a reasonable attitude for neurophysiologists to take in their studies; but it does not dispose of the question of consciousness. In fact Wolfgang Schlote of the Institute for Brain Research at the University of Tübingen comments on Eccles's statement:

'And yet consciousness, the capacity for conscious experience, which has only gradually appeared in evolutionary development and the development of individual forms of life, and which we use in most though not all of our actions, must be implicated in the way of functioning of that multi-cellular organ, the central nervous system.'

17

Dark-Room of Nightmares

It was dark and quiet in the narrow cell. No sound penetrated the strong walls. There was not the slightest glimmer of light to relieve what the subject later called 'the deepest darkness I have ever experienced'. He was a student at Princeton University, New Jersey, and was one of many who spent ninety-six hours in a room only ten feet square in area, almost completely filled by a bed. As instructed by Jack Vernon, the director of the experiment, they lay on the bed as still as possible and stared into the darkness when they were not sleeping. They might only leave the bed when they wanted to take food from a refrigerator or use the toilets—in an anteroom which was also totally sound-proof and in complete darkness.

They had all volunteered for an experiment which promised a few lazy days for good pay. They were very ready to expose themselves to the darkness and silence in the 'dark-room' through which Vernon and his colleagues at Princeton were trying to find out how people behave when cut off from the outside world. What does the brain do if the flow of messages which are usually transmitted continuously by the sense organs is all of a sudden strongly reduced for days at a time? How does it react to a drastic limitation of input? This method of psychological research, known as sensory deprivation, revealed a considerable potential for opportunities of manipulating the human brain.

The phrase 'sensory deprivation' is of course somewhat exaggerated. In no experiment have researchers succeeded in completely 'switching off' all sense organs for a period and so denying the brain all sensory stimuli. But however incomplete the efforts may have been to block the flow of communications from the outside world, the effects were impressive enough. 'Never before', said Vernon, 'has a person been so completely dependent on himself (and to discover how little he has left then can be a terrifying experience).'

In this state the brain is grateful for any stimulation. It is a state which offers the best chances for brain-washing.

Brain manipulation without current or chemicals

That it does not need the direct action of electrical or chemical stimuli to manipulate a brain is no new discovery. Over thousands of years indirect methods have been used and have proved very effective. Often they have been misused; for their misuse is much easier to organise than brain manipulation by electrical or chemical stimuli, and these methods lead with far greater probability, at least in the short term, to the results desired by the manipulators.

We all manipulate brains, of course, by indirect (psychological) means; and our own brains are manipulated from childhood on. We are induced to behave in particular ways, and we in turn influence the behaviour of our children. The young are exposed to the form of brain manipulation called education; they learn from the society in which they grow up. But many of the norms of behaviour and attitudes instilled into the young do not have anything like the absolute validity which educators might sometimes claim for them. Obviously the rules on how one behaves, what one may say, do and think, are different in different societies and they change with time. One recent minor illustration of the time-change is the wearing of very long hair by young men, considered highly effeminate not so long ago, but for a decade a fashion almost universally accepted in many Western countries by the young of both sexes, even if still disapproved of by many older people. The 'generation gap', of course, is no novelty either.

Many parents through the ages have tried to force their children into habits familiar to them (the parents) or to the parents' own taste. This may be called brain manipulation in the bad sense, and however well meant, it is harmful and often counter-productive. When the young recognise the irrelevance or apparent stupidity of some of the maxims thrust upon them, they are inclined to doubt the value of even sensible advice or instruction, and in their rebellion make the parents even more insistent on their own rightness. The conflict between the generations becomes grooved in a vicious circle.

Far more menacing for the individual are the measures of tyrannical rulers and the officials of dictatorial systems who want to make the brains of their subjects obedient. In all ages, again, rulers have tried to reinforce their power by rewards for the submissive and severe punishments for the rebellious. When religious or political ideology is involved, there are subtler methods of exerting influence, so that the autocrats' subjects not only accept absolute rule, but are also induced to believe in the creeds which the autocrat has declared obligatory.

For centuries the Inquisitors hunted for contemporaries who strayed from the exact doctrine which could alone bring salvation. In the name of Christ millions of heretics were hurled into prison, tortured and burned. Men who did not feel bound by any legal rules organised trials which had as their chief aim to make the accused confess their sins, real or alleged, against the orthodox line. The pressure was psychological as well as physical: the refractory were threatened with confiscation of their property, disinheritance of their families and grave disadvantages for their children and descendants. Only submissiveness could lead to a lenient outcome of the trial; the humbled sinner had to prove himself worthy of his judges' indulgence by vehement protestation and demonstration of belief.

In our era the Nazi and Communist leaders reproduced on a more massive scale, with the benefit of their totalitarian powers, the inhuman methods of brain manipulation from the Middle Ages. But in contrast to the Nazis, who were not interested in 'converting' heretics or scapegoats, Stalin readopted the procedure of the Inquisition: his henchmen extorted lengthy confessions of guilt from prominent victims, even when they had no chance of surviving their ideological error, misjudgment of a situation, or difference of opinion with a more powerful official. In the late nineteen-thirties the world watched with amazement the show-trials in Moscow, where dozens of top communists, with certain death before their eyes, denounced their own treason and sabotage, giving details which in some cases were later exposed as clearly inventions.

How were intelligent people induced even to make up stories justifying their own death sentence? Torture, still the most terrifying means of brain manipulation, may make the victims do or say anything just to have it stop. The readiness to confess may be increased by threats to liquidate the families of the accused. But Arthur Koestler, former supporter of communism and therefore familiar with its methods, has shown convincingly in his novel dealing with the Moscow trials, *Darkness at Noon*, that skilful manipulation can even without torture develop this readiness, which can then be demonstrated more safely in court.

The hero of the novel, People's Commissar Rubachov, who has fallen into disfavour, is softened up by alternating friendly and harsh treatment, by day-long interrogations and breaks for reflection. His inquisitors charge him with inconsistency and confront him with wrong decisions he has made. They remind him of things he once said himself, though in a different situation; of his duty to the Party, which is always right, now too when it demands confessions from him. Rubachov knows the liquidation machinery, he knows he cannot escape it. Finally he is consoled by the thought that he can render a last service to the Party, for which he has worked all his life, by making the confessions demanded of him.

However these confessions were achieved in Soviet Russia and during the post-war decade in the countries of Eastern Europe dominated by Russia, the initiators and their henchmen established a horrifying example of brain manipulation.

Chinese brain-washing

The Chinese communists were equally thorough, perhaps even more so, in their methods of securing ideological orthodoxy. In 1949, soon after the 'People's Liberation Army' had occupied the last remains of the Chinese mainland, the new rulers started on a ruthless programme for the political 're-education' of all who were suspected of a bourgeois attitude because of their non-communist origins. Mao Tse-tung and his supporters considered such re-education essential before former enemies or the indifferent could become members of the new society. In the United States the phrase 'brain-washing' was coined for the Chinese variant of brain manipulation—a new term for an old evil. It was not only the Chinese who were exposed to such brain-washing, but also Europeans and Americans living in China and arrested by the communists and soldiers from America and other countries taken prisoner during the Korean war.

The tactics of brain-washing consisted in isolating the individual and destroying his connection with anybody not a communist. The conviction was then drilled into him that his behaviour and ideas were wrong and that his salvation could lie only in rendering loyal service to the Communist Party and obeying it unconditionally.

Prisons again proved valuable manipulation centres. The prisoners were separated from friends and relations, cut off from information sources and removed from all the things which would otherwise have occupied their day. Rules were imposed designed to humiliate them, to which they had to submit without protest. Eating, sleeping, washing and even excreting had to be carried out according to a strict daily routine. To do anything without the warder's permission was forbidden. The prisoners had to approach the warder with bowed head and eyes lowered. Neglect of the rules was punished with deprivation of food, continual disturbance of sleep or being put in fetters.

They were told that they must make progress in the learning process if they wanted to win back their freedom. Cell-mates at a more advanced stage of the brain-washing would try to distinguish themselves by converting those who were still of little faith. At the advanced stage prisoners could attend daily courses in communist doctrine. But more important were the discussions, in which the re-education pupils were compelled to apply the doctrine to their whole lives, confess how greatly they had formerly sinned against it, and to repent of their errors. Thus prepared, they could finally face their trial, at which they received a lenient sentence for the crimes confessed. If they survived this too, they were considered manipulated enough to be acknowledged as members of the new society. The whole procedure might take six months, but also four years or more.

The American prisoners from the Korean war were subjected to a far less intensive 'brain-washing'; which caused all the greater shock in America when it became known that thirteen per cent of the United States soldiers had 'collaborated' with the Chinese. Patriots deplored the small powers of resistance shown by the 'traitors' and saw it as a sign of growing softness in the American character. Today it is recognised by the press and even by the military that isolation, interrogations, continual pressure and other features of brain-washing can break the will of even the toughest people. The question, declared the Princeton psychiatrist, Bryant M. Wedge, who studied repatriated United States prisoners of war from Korea, 'is not one of the American character, but of the nature of the human mind itself'.

Effects of sensory deprivation

Clearly, the brain obeys laws which limit the powers of resistance to psychological methods of brain manipulation. The investigations on sensory deprivation helped greatly towards the recognition that this was the case. They were initiated in the early 'fifties by psychologist Donald Hebb at McGill University in Montreal, with sponsorship from the Canadian Defence Research Board. Like their colleagues in the United States, Canada's service chiefs felt uneasy about how susceptible the Korean prisoners had proved to brain-washing. They were also depressed by a phenomenon which weakened their military preparedness: radar observers, radio operators and other specialists who had to carry out monotonous work for hours on end suddenly became the victims of strange delusions. They saw on the radar screen objects that were not there at all, or declared they had heard messages which nobody had transmitted.

Hebb could not, of course, subject to torture those who

volunteered for his experiments! But as in the Chinese 're-education' process solitary confinement had played an important part, it looked a promising idea merely to isolate the volunteers from their usual environment and to cut them off as completely as possible from impressions which the sense organs were normally transmitting all the time to the brain. He also hoped that such experiments would provide an explanation for the breakdowns of the radar observers and radio operators.

The student volunteers could leave the solitary confinement room at any time, but this would mean that the experiment was ended for them. Their single cells were neither dark nor sound-proof, but Hebb curtailed their sensations of sight, touch and hearing: they had to wear close-fitting spectacles with frosted-glass lenses, gloves and also cardboard handcuffs; and they were deafened by the noise from the air-conditioning plant.

Pay was generous: twenty dollars a day simply for doing nothing, at a time when the dollar bought far more than it does today. Despite that, some of the students found the new experience so intolerable that they broke off the experiment on the first day. They complained above all of no longer being able to think coherently. With others it had to be broken off abruptly later on, following sudden outbursts of rage or fits of terror at the thought of staying in the room a minute longer. Those who stuck it out till the end of the experiment (up to six days) manifested various peculiarities, including hallucinations and delusions. They saw squirrels, heard music, felt they had two bodies or thought their heads had been detached from their bodies.

Hebb has shown, in fact, that a treatment less severe than torture is calculated to put the human brain in a condition which it finds intolerable and which could successfully condition it for a brain-washing.

Soon other researchers, including Vernon at Princeton, undertook studies on the effects of sensory deprivation.

Vernon's subjects in the dark-room did not even see diffused light (as Hebb's did), and all they could hear was the soft hiss of their own breathing. He dispensed, however, with the handcuffs, so they could feel more than Hebb's subjects. Vernon wrote a book about his experiments (which were backed by the United States Army), in which he too showed the part which sensory deprivation could play in brain-washing.

What does a person feel like when his brain in the dark-room suffers from lack of input? Most of the subjects at Princeton soon realised that they had greatly underestimated the ordeal to which they had voluntarily exposed themselves. They were to spend from forty-eight to ninety-six hours in the dark-room under the conditions of sensory deprivation. Most of them went into the experiment very readily, seeing it as a welcome opportunity, for twenty-five dollars a day, to think about their work or personal problems. But very few were satisfied afterwards with the results of their thinking: as with Hebb's subjects, most complained that after a while they could no longer concentrate, that their thoughts went round in a circle or that they kept getting stuck at the same thought.

Soon after lying down in the dark-room, they all started by falling into a long deep sleep. The psychologists who had expected that the volunteers would be excited in the unfamiliar surroundings and that sleep was one thing they would not do, felt this was a waste of precious experiment time, and tried beginning the experiment in the morning when the students would have had their full night's sleep. But even then they went to sleep just as soon. They were escaping from the monotony, Vernon concluded. 'It was a very effective technique, but it was not a voluntary action. They did not say: "This is boring, I want to go to sleep." . . . Sleep came quickly and automatically.'

Almost all subjects considerably underrated the time they had slept. One student slept nineteen hours at a stretch (a

microphone stuck in the cell transmitted his deep breathing),
but later declared that he had only had a short sleep, no
more than two hours.

Most of the subjects survived the first day in their
confinement without difficulty, mainly because they slept
so well. Then the situation began to become critical for
many of them. They had all had their sleep out, and the
brain started to suffer from lack of stimulating messages.
Before the second day was over, every fifth subject had
pressed the 'panic button', a bell within easy reach with
which they could call Vernon or one of his assistants to
break off the experiment.

The students gave various reasons for their surrender.
Some were tormented by intolerable nightmares, others
suffered from headaches or stomach-aches. One gave up
because he 'could no longer sleep', another because he
imagined he had gone blind. Several subjects indeed had the
same delusion, though others convinced themselves they
were not blind by hitting themselves lightly on the eyes and
finding with relief that this still made them 'see stars'. One
subject who pressed the panic button after thirty-six hours
had reached the conclusion that he was being underpaid.
Evidently, said Vernon, all his attempts to adapt himself to
the conditions of sensory deprivation had gone adrift.

Of those who left the room prematurely, one in three
wanted to continue the experiment directly he got outside;
this was not allowed, as it would have falsified the results.
But quite a number said straight out that they never
wanted to go through anything like it again. Vernon
commented: 'One cannot avoid thinking about what
happens to a person when imprisonment is forcibly continued
as, say, in a brain-washing situation. It would probably
be relatively simple to bring that person to change his
attitude, to sign confessions or do almost anything else to
be released.'

Vernon demonstrated in an impressive manner how

greatly the subjects needed sense stimuli which offered distraction. In one series of experiments he installed in the cell a peep-show which subjects could switch on and off when they liked. What they saw was nothing very exciting: two circles and a line faintly limned against a dark background. In normal circumstances the students would have given such a pattern no more than a fleeting glance. An automatic recording device showed that those enclosed in the darkness paid it far more attention. Obviously their brains clamoured so strongly for excitement that even this simple pattern seemed an attraction.

On average the subjects looked at the picture for three minutes in 72 hours. Asked afterwards about their interest in it, all of them said they had looked at the peep-show less often than they had really done: say only 5 times instead of 32, only 25 times instead of 121. Apparently it was embarrassing for them to admit having spent so much time looking at so uninteresting a picture.

Vernon and his colleagues had long been searching for criteria which would enable them to predict which subjects would stick the experiment out and which would break it off prematurely. The peep-show proved an important aid to such a prognosis, and soon divided them up. The students who gave in, regardless of the reasons they offered for doing so, spent on average fifteen times as long at the peep-show as those who went through the whole experiment.

The psychologists regularly observed some striking effects from the sensory deprivation. Almost all the subjects lost several pounds in weight, although they had plenty to eat (3000 calories a day) and scarcely moved. After the experiment their reactions had slowed up, and their sensitivity to pain had increased.

But certainly the most important effect as regards brainwashing is the greater receptiveness to propaganda. Donald Hebb at Montreal succeeded in making students believe in poltergeists, when they had been thoroughly sceptical before the experiment about there being such spirits. He simply had the isolated subjects listen to a tape on which a very convincing voice gave alleged proofs for the existence of poltergeists.

At Princeton a colleague of Vernon's, Peter Suedfeld, made a number of students into admirers of Turkey. He got them to answer a questionnaire before they entered the dark-room, to establish whether they had any special interest in or liking for that country; none of them had. After they had spent twenty-four hours in the dark-room, he played them a tape with a propaganda talk in praise of Turkey. A second questionnaire revealed that this primitive form of instruction had been effective: the students now felt very friendly towards Turkey. With a group of students, however, who had not been in the dark-room, the propaganda had little or no effect.

'The enclosed individual', Vernon commented, 'experiences terrible monotony and boredom so that he actively seeks almost any form of stimulation. If for any reason we had the desire to develop a superior system of brain-washing, we could use to our advantage this search for stimulation.'

What such a 'superior system' might be like, he illustrated by an example: assuming a Protestant were to be converted to Islam, one might first expose him for four days to sensory deprivation under strict conditions, and then, when his brain was pining for stimulation, show him two switches which he could activate at will. If he pressed Switch A, he could hear a thirty-second talk in favour of the Protestant faith. By pressing Switch B he could hear propaganda for Islam. But there was an important difference between the two switches. A provided the same talk every time, given by the same voice; B offered different talks by different voices. 'In this way,' says Vernon, 'the monotony of the sensory deprivation would be connected with the monotony of the continuously repeated Protestant talk, and the wish for excitement would lead to Switch B being chosen. . . . We have then made this individual listen to our propaganda by his own choice. If we induce him to listen to it, we can also convince him of it by drafting our propaganda cleverly enough.'

No one has yet washed brains as elegantly as this. It is certainly a horrifying thought that under suitable conditions, without even the need for a long and complicated treatment, our brains will choose just what the 'washers' want us to absorb. There may, however, be one small consolation in a brutal world, where large sections of mankind are continually falling under the sway of fanatical autocrats who use any means to enforce the loyalty and orthodoxy of their subjects. Perhaps their classical procedure will be superseded if Vernon's suggestion, at present only hypothetical, is ever realised: sensory deprivation might replace long imprisonment and torture, deprivation of food and sleep, devices to humiliate, and pitiless interrogations. It is a far from cheering prospect, but while such ruthless regimes exist, the reduction in violence would at least be some improvement for their victims.

18

Sleep and Dreams

'When it is night,' declared the great neurophysiologist Sir
Charles Sherrington, 'the lights go out in the brain too. Only
isolated points flicker in remote regions; most of the brain
is at rest in the darkness till sleep is over and a myriad lights
flash on again. It is as if the Milky Way entered upon some
cosmic dance. Swiftly the head mass becomes an enchanted
loom, where millions of flashing shuttles weave a dissolving
pattern, always a meaningful pattern though never an
abiding one.'

The lyrical words of the British Nobel prize-winner now
have only literary value: there is plenty of light in the brain
while we sleep. Sherrington, who died in 1952, could not
know this. Only a year after his death a discovery was made
which started a boom in sleep research, fundamentally
altering our ideas about sleep.

Today, in dozens of specially equipped sleep laboratories,
measuring instruments are attached night after night to test
subjects healthy and sick, and all phases of their sleep are
watched. Researchers intrude into their dreams, and do not

for a single moment leave the slumbering brain, which has switched off its consciousness, unmonitored by the instruments. A single research team, directed by Uroš J. Jovanović in the nerve and pediatric clinic of the University of Würzburg, in close co-operation with two psychiatric clinics in Zagreb, has in two years registered and assessed 1300 nights' sleep.

For thousands of years philosophers, scientists and poets have been concerned with sleep:

> Sleep that knits up the ravell'd sleave of care,
> The death of each day's life, sore labour's bath,
> Balm of hurt minds, great nature's second course,
> Chief nourisher in life's feast.

Aristotle taught that it was designed to contribute towards the preservation of life; Freud remarked: 'Our relationship to the world into which we came so unwillingly seems to include an inability to tolerate it without interruption.' But as to the causes of sleep, even the most distinguished scientists could only produce hypotheses and speculations.

It was said to be produced, for instance, by a drop in the blood supply to the brain. Or, we were made tired by blocking of the central nervous system, or the agglomeration of 'exhaustion substances' which took place in the waking state and had to be reduced in sleep. Or, sleep ensued when brain cells contracted their dendrites and so broke the connections with each other; or, when an innate protective instinct found it best to preserve the organism from exhaustion. But there were very few precise findings to accompany the theories. The way into the mysterious realm, in which we spend a third of our lives unconscious, seemed barred to research.

The imaginations of philosophers, poets and priests, doctors and finally other scientists as well, were excited even more strongly by sleep's accompanying phenomenon—

dreams. Though often impressive for their bizarre content, dream experiences usually disappeared quickly from memory, and therefore faced researchers with difficult problems in their attempts to gain exact knowledge. In his early days Freud, the most famous of dream interpreters, complained that there had not yet been achieved 'the development of a foundation of confirmed results so that the immediate successors in research could then have built on to them. Every new authority tackles the same problems again and as if starting again from the beginning.'

In his work *The Interpretation of Dreams*, published in 1900, Freud was convinced he had solved the age-old problem. He believed that the sleeper in his dreams allowed wishes to be registered which could not be fulfilled in real life— mostly wishes which the dreamer did not dare admit to himself. The fulfilment of 'improper' wishes was therefore encoded in apparently meaningless or absurd dream images. So dreams 'defused' conflict situations which would make people sleepless. For the founder of psychoanalysis, dreams were in this sense the guardians of sleep.

But like his countless predecessors in dream interpretation, Freud could only speculate about the nature of dreaming on the basis of shreds of dreams which happened to be remembered and subjective reports that could scarcely be checked.

Half a century later Hans Winterstein, the German researcher into sleep and dreams, confessed that there was total uncertainty concerning the basic questions of his special research field. 'The reproduction of a dream of whose existence we know', he wrote in 1953, 'causes us the greatest difficulties as it is. The actual length of the dream period . . . cannot so far be at all established. Deep sleep is dreamless, say some, and the dream is only a phenomenon of the transition from the sleeping to the waking state. We always dream, say others, but we cannot remember dreams, because they leave no trace in our memory.'

Rapid eye movements: the key to dreaming

The possibility of experimental research on dreams was revealed about this time by the investigation of a phenomenon which at first appeared of rather secondary importance: the movement of people's eyeballs when they sleep. These studies found the key to the realm of dreams, and their results proved the starting-point for an extraordinarily fruitful development in sleep research.

Two researchers at the University of Chicago, Nathaniel Kleitman and his colleague, Eugene Aserinsky, noticed with sleeping children that the eyeballs under the closed lids sometimes rolled violently to and fro. This observation was not new. The eye movements conspicuous at the lids can be recognised by anyone who watches a sleeper carefully and continuously. But Aserinsky now set about registering these movements.

To catch every eyeball movement, he stuck near the children's eyes 'antennae', which were connected by thin wires to an automatic registering instrument, an electro-oculograph. An assistant recorded exactly the movements of the eyes. The results showed that with every child periods in which the eyes moved rapidly set in several times a night. Investigations on adults revealed the same phenomenon.

Aserinsky's chief, Kleitman, had the idea that the eye movements might have something to do with dreams. To give substance to this suspicion, he woke test subjects at different times: sometimes during the eye-rolling, sometimes in the phases when the eyes were at rest. Soon he saw his hypothesis confirmed: if the subjects were woken during the eye-rolling, they almost always reported on a dream they had just had; if they were woken in a phase when the eyes were at rest, they could not as a rule remember any dream.

With William Dement, another member of his team, Kleitman worked out an extensive dream-research programme. For a few dollars a night volunteers slept and dreamt in the 'sleep-lab', allowed themselves to be wrenched from slumber several times a night in order to say whether they had just dreamt and, if so, what. A tape-recorder in the sleep-room took down their accounts of dreams.

In this way the Chicago researchers obtained the first sure knowledge about dreams. Many popular ideas, which till then could be neither proved nor refuted, turned out to be wrong. Dement and Kleitman established, for instance, that in good health there is no one who seldom or never dreams; on the contrary, everybody dreams four or five times every night. Even subjects who had declared they never dreamed, described their dreams on tape after being torn from sleep during the eye-rolling period.

Dreams do not last only a few seconds, as even many researchers had formerly believed; their length varies between eight minutes and half an hour. Altogether dreaming takes place during about a fifth of the night's sleep.

Dement tried to manipulate the content of dreams by squirting his volunteer sleepers with water or plying them with noise. It proved that such external stimuli, like internal causes—thirst, full bladder, etc.—did sometimes influence the dream's content, but (contrary to a widespread view) never caused a dream. It is also not true that women dream more often than men and passionate people more often than phlegmatic people! It is the case, however, that many people are better than others at remembering their dreams. Another idea refuted was that restless movements in sleep indicate that the sleeper is dreaming. He is more likely to be lying still when dreaming. He will move before the dream, rather as people at a theatre shift about in their seats before the performance starts, but sit quite still once the curtain has gone up. Sleep-walkers do not make their nightly excursions during dream phases.

Two quite different types of sleep

The sleep associated with dreams was called REM (Rapid Eye Movement) sleep. But extensive investigations at Chicago, and soon elsewhere as well, showed that it differed from other sleep not only in its eye movements and dreams. The transition from one phase of sleep to another was clearly recognisable on the EEG (electroencephalograph), which registered variations of tension in the brain.

Such variations in electrical potential can comfortably be recorded through the top of the skull by the recording devices available today. Electroencephalography, developed in the 'twenties by the German psychiatrist Hans Berger at the University of Jena, is an important investigative process which gives much information on the activity of healthy and sick brains. In many clinics and research institutes the twitching pencils of EEGs register thousands of miles of differing wave-like forms in complex patterns—which can then be analysed.

The transition from the dreamless sleep phase to REM sleep is also associated with a number of other characteristic changes. Breathing becomes faster and more irregular, blood pressure increases. The blood supply to the cerebral cortex also goes up, often far above the level measured in the waking state. The muscles relax, although with men the penis stiffens regularly and persistently; with women blood flows to the clitoris, which leads to a rise in temperature; this does not sink again till the end of the REM sleep. The reactions taking place all night at the sex organs without our knowledge, astonishing in their extent, were exactly and continuously recorded for the first time by Jovanović in Würzburg with special instruments registering automatically.

From all this it is established that there is nothing uniform about sleep. The unconsciousness in which we spend our nights is composed of two basically different states which succeed each other several times in the course of a night.

'The period of rapid eye movement', declared Dement, one of the sleep research pioneers, 'is a special state of being.' Our lives consist not only of waking and sleeping but of three phases: waking, normal sleep, REM sleep.

But the course of sleep even in the period between the REM phases is irregular. By the marking of the EEG lines sleep researchers distinguish five stages from sleep-inclined mood (Stage 1) to deep sleep (Stage 4) and Stage 1 REM. The deeper the sleep, the more difficult the sleeper is to awaken. Still stronger waking stimuli are needed, of course, in REM sleep, although the EEG curves in this phase of sleep are rather like those of the waking state.

So we swing in sleep not only between normal and REM sleep but also on the waves of varying depths of sleep. We spend only a small part of our night's sleep at Stage 1— between 11.2 and 19.5 per cent of the whole sleeping time (as Jovanović and his team discovered).

The observation that the sleep of mammals, and to a lesser degree of birds, is full of REM phases like man's, suggested that they too dream in their way (although it is hard to imagine the secret wishes which according to Freud are fulfilled in their dreams!). The characteristics of REM sleep were also shown in new-born babies. Babies, in fact, spend far more of their much longer sleeping time in REM sleep—about half of it. New-born kittens, rats and rabbits have exclusively REM sleep. What should the kittens dream of? Clearly the idea adopted at first, that dreams are the most important feature of REM sleep, was no longer tenable: modern sleep research, which started as dream research, did not remain at that.

Sleep centres in the brain stem

Apart from the fact that the researchers woke their volunteers several times a night to question them about dreams, the exciting results of sleep research so far described were achieved simply by observing and measuring processes of life taking place normally. Such purely recording investigations could not answer many basic questions about sleep.

What happens in the brain when we sleep? What centres are responsible for the control of sleep? What substances are involved? Why do we need to sleep at all, and for what do we use the two kinds of sleep? If researchers wanted to find answers to questions like these, they could not confine themselves to observing people and animals in sleep. They had to experiment with brains.

We have already seen something of the pioneering experiments, starting in the 'twenties, by W. R. Hess, the Swiss physiologist who was awarded the Nobel Prize in 1949 (see Chapter 7). Among the discoveries he reported from stimulating cats' brains with electrical current was that if the stimuli were applied to a certain region of the thalamus, the cats began to blink and after a while went to sleep.

Other researchers, however, recorded the same reaction to electrical stimulation of other parts of the brain, certain points in the cerebrum and the cerebellum, in the hypothalamus and the brain stem. That a definite centre actively controls sleep could not be concluded from these confusing results. Assessment of them was also made harder by the fact that even without brain stimulation cats sleep for sixty to seventy per cent of their lives.

If sleep is more than 'exhausted wakefulness', if it is a phenomenon which actively sets in and is not characterised merely by the absence of another state, then proof was needed that test animals could be robbed of their sleep by elimination of particular parts of the brain. A group of Italian researchers, directed by Giuseppe Moruzzi, succeeded in producing this proof in the late 'fifties.

He and his team severed the brain stem of cats below the mid-brain reticular activation system (see Chapter 8). In consequence the cats slept only twenty per cent of the time.

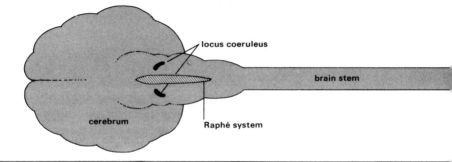

locus coeruleus

brain stem

cerebrum

Raphé system

In the brain of cats, centres were discovered which control sleep. These centres are in the brain stem. The front part of the Raphé system (left in drawing) is responsible for 'normal sleep', the tail part and the two bean-shaped 'blue places' known as locus coeruleus regulate dream sleep.

During the rest of it they regarded their surroundings with wide-awake eyes, and the EEG of the cerebral cortices showed the typical form of the waking state. The result of this experiment left no doubt that the incision stopped centres in the lower parts of the brain stem from exerting sleep-promoting influence on the brain.

The researchers had thus defined the region of the brain where the search for sleep centres would have to be made. Since then it has been possible to find out the brain structures which have to work together in order to produce sleep. A 'chemistry of sleep' is also emerging, and has already developed far enough for scientists to be able at choice to switch normal or REM sleep on or off through particular substances. We owe important discoveries about the anatomy and chemistry of sleep to the French sleep researcher Michel Jouvet and his colleagues at the University of Lyon.

A long narrow zone exactly on the centre line of the brain stem which is called the 'Raphé system' (the word *raphé*, derived from the Greek, means 'seam'), was identified by Jouvet as an important sleep centre. When he and his colleagues destroyed eighty to ninety per cent of this part of the brain stem in cats, the cats did not sleep at all for three or four days. Later they found some sleep, but only slept for ten per cent of the time at most, and the EEG showed only normal sleep; they did not have any more REM sleep. But if a smaller part of the Raphé system was destroyed, part of the capacity for sleep remained intact. If the cats slept over fifteen per cent of the time, they also had some REM sleep.

In operations where only smaller parts of the Raphé system were destroyed, the researchers discovered that there was a release mechanism at the tail end of the Raphé system, nearest to the spinal cord. For when only this part of the Raphé system was affected, all they observed in the cats was a reduced quota of REM sleep. Operations on the front part of the Raphé system, on the other hand, impaired normal sleep, but scarcely affected REM sleep. Some of the cats were no longer capable of normal sleep at all but got through as much REM sleep as before the operation.

The caudal (tail) part of the Raphé system is not the only centre which controls REM sleep. A part is also played by two small bean-shaped centres in the brain stem to the right and left of the Raphé system. They look blue and are therefore called *locus coeruleus* (blue place). When researchers destroyed the locus coeruleus the cats lost their REM sleep.

Manipulating sleep mechanisms

Jouvet and his colleagues succeeded in proving that two substances—which we have met before—are indispensable for sleep: serotonin and noradrenalin. Both function as transmitters in the synaptic gaps. It was explained in Chapter 14 why psychiatrists believe that lack of these substances in the relevant synaptic gaps leads to depressions. In this connection it is interesting that patients with depressions often suffer also from tormenting sleep troubles.

There is another striking connection: reserpine, a drug for treating depression seldom used today, can lead to a condition which looks very like a depression, and it too may banish sleep for a long time. In experiments on cats, reserpine suppressed normal sleep for twelve hours, and REM sleep for as much as twenty-four hours. This psychoactive drug reduced the amount of serotonin and noradrenalin in the brain. If it does that, Jouvet reflected, one should be able to remove the reserpine effect by helping to restore in the brain a higher amount of serotonin and noradrenalin. Since these two substances do not pass the blood-brain-barrier, it was no good injecting them into the circulation. So the researchers injected into animals certain substances which are their precursors and which enter the brain without difficulty. The expected effect promptly occurred. A serotonin precursor, a substance called 5-hydroxytryptophan, quickly sent to sleep the cats treated with reserpine, while the noradrenalin precursor, dihydroxyphenylalanine, specifically gave rise to REM sleep.

Then Jouvet tried to lower separately the concentration of serotonin and noradrenalin. He first used a substance called p-chlorophenylalanine, which inhibits the forming of serotonin. He injected this inhibiting substance into cats. For twenty-four hours nothing happened: the cats slept as usual for a good deal of the time. But then sleep troubles set in. Between thirty and sixty hours after the beginning of the experiment the sleep-loving animals found no sleep at all. After this long break sleep gradually started again. They did not sleep their normal amount till two hundred hours after the beginning of the experiment.

But even at the peak of their sleeplessness Jouvet could neutralise at any time the effect of the inhibiting substance: by an injection of the serotonin element 5-hydroxytryptophan. After one injection, containing only a few milligrams of the substance, the cats slept from six to ten hours. Then the effect of the sleep-inhibiting substance won the upper hand again.

Jouvet also interfered in the noradrenalin make-up. Various inhibiting substances could be used for that. They did not lead to sleeplessness but exclusively suppressed REM sleep. Supposing that cats dream, these cats, after injection of a substance inhibiting noradrenalin, were robbed of their dreams.

In a comprehensive report on his experiments, Jouvet wrote that they showed very convincingly that 'sleep mechanisms can be manipulated at will'. They have led him to the following idea of the significance of serotonin and noradrenalin for sleep: serotonin is indispensable for normal sleep and is also a prerequisite for the development of REM sleep; but before REM sleep can actually take place, an adequate concentration of noradrenalin is needed as well. These biochemical beliefs, however, are not by any means universally accepted.

Swedish researchers established the connection between chemical and anatomical discoveries in sleep research. They found that the cells of the Raphé system, whose destruction causes insomnia, were rich in serotonin. The locus coeruleus, on the other hand, whose surgical elimination banished REM sleep, contained a good deal of noradrenalin.

Informative as these results are, they do not explain, it is true, why we have to sleep at all, why we cannot—like bull-frogs and crocodiles, for instance—do without sleep altogether.

Sleep deprivation tests

Everyone knows from his own experience, of course, how hard it is, after a night with little sleep, to perform work requiring attention and concentration. Anybody who spends more than one night not sleeping soon comes near the point where he feels he just cannot go on. So deprivation of sleep is one of the methods of torture by which brain-washers try to extort secrets or enforce loyalty to the party line. Obviously we need sleep for the brain to retain its efficiency; but that is no explanation, only a statement of fact.

In order to find out more about sleep, scientists have

repeatedly deprived volunteers of sleep for a period, either completely or partially, and during that period carried out observations, measurements and tests. In the Würzburg sleep sanatorium attempts were made to keep two students awake continuously for five days, which at the end of the experiment did not prove wholly practical: as the EEG showed, they could scarcely be kept from going to sleep on their feet with their eyes open. After the experiment was broken off, one student slept for twelve hours, the other for sixteen. Both said they had completely recovered after this sleep, which showed a much increased proportion of Stage 3 and 4 sleep; later on they made up more on their REM sleep.

What effect did the sleeplessness have during the experiment? In the first forty-eight hours the students behaved fairly normally. The observers noticed only a slight tendency to mistrust and edginess. After the third day without sleep they became very irritable and quarrelsome, their mistrust grew. At the same time they became so nervous that they started at every noise. Sometimes the world swam before their eyes, and they saw people and pictures distorted. But the whole time they were fully aware of their situation.

Various tests they had to carry out revealed, right till the end of the experiment, an astonishing efficiency for simple problems. With more complicated ones, demanding adaptability, concentration and sustained attention, a considerable drop in performance was shown after only twenty-one hours—a result of great interest for drivers. The Würzburg sleep researchers were particularly impressed by the fact that their tired subjects were inclined at quite an early stage to over-rate their capacities.

The need for dream sleep

So the subjects had to make up their quota of dream sleep

as well as the deep sleep on stages 3 and 4. But what is the purpose of this dream sleep? It was clearly 'invented' only at an advanced stage in the natural evolution of brains. What does it mean for the brains of mammals and man? Researchers have tried to answer the question by deliberately depriving animals and men of the REM sleep for a time; but the results have proved disappointing.

One method consisted in always waking up subjects whenever EEG and eye movements showed that the sleepers were starting to dream. This happened twenty-two times in the first disturbed night and afterwards even more often. In 1960 William Dement, who carried out those experiments, reported dramatic effects: his subjects had shown signs of personality change and suffered from hallucinations. But in later experimental series he did not find the observations confirmed, and retracted the results first published as mistaken. One thing which is established is that after the loss of REM sleep, that loss is made up.

Jouvet could not report any more exciting results from stopping cats falling into REM sleep for weeks at a time. He would put a cat on a small, low platform in the middle of some water. It could sit comfortably on the platform and enjoy its normal sleep in the position characteristic of cats. But directly it fell into REM sleep and its muscles relaxed so that it lay on its side, its head came into contact with the water, and it woke up. Even when the REM sleep had been suppressed in this way for three weeks, Jouvet could establish no worse consequences than a slightly accelerated heart-beat.

Yet something important must have been missed through the suspension of REM sleep. For directly the cats could leave the platform and were allowed to have REM sleep again, they had it intensively. For days the proportion of REM sleep in the whole sleeping time was up to sixty per cent instead of the usual fifteen. After three weeks' suspension of REM sleep it took about ten days before the need to catch up on it had been satisfied. So REM sleep seems to be less important for cats than for man, even though its rôle in promoting their well-being has so far been just as little explained.

We could be more satisfied with the finding that deprivation of REM sleep causes no conspicuous damage, if the question were not of practical importance for many people because of the use of psychoactive drugs. All drugs affecting the brain—narcotics and tranquillisers, drugs for the mentally sick and intoxicating or 'trip' drugs—influence the pattern of sleep phases and stages. Most of these substances, for instance barbiturates, alcohol, heroin, stimulants and tranquillisers, drastically reduce the REM sleep (although it goes back to normal as the taker adapts to these drugs). We cannot dismiss out of hand the suspicion that this limitation of REM sleep produces subtle changes, which may have very serious effects if the drugs are used over a long period. The development of new narcotics and drugs for the mentally sick now includes investigations of their influence on the quality of sleep as part of the standard programme.

The brain reacts to chemical suppression of REM sleep no differently from its reaction to interference with the natural conditions through constant waking; it makes up the REM sleep as soon as it can, and even gets itself more REM sleep than it would have had in normal circumstances. Ian Oswald of the Department of Psychiatry at Edinburgh

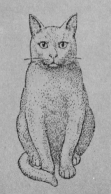
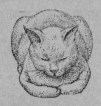
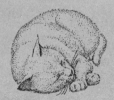

Cats sleep a lot; their position shows whether they are in normal sleep (centre) or paradoxical sleep (right)

University found that, after narcotic poisoning, a few shots of heroin or an overdose of librium, the proportion of REM sleep is at first strikingly reduced and then increased for two months; during this period twice as much REM sleep is 'made up' as was missed.

This neutralising effect is also shown with new-born children when the mothers have been treated during pregnancy with phenothiazines, antidotes to schizophrenia. Normally the proportion of the baby's REM sleep, at first very high, slowly goes down from day to day. With the children of women treated with a phenothiazine however, the proportion of REM sleep immediately goes up still further.

Why must we sleep?

The very comprehensive investigations of modern sleep research have still not answered the question as to the purpose of sleep but there are theories. One comes from Ian Oswald of Edinburgh. To summarise his theory, it says that normal sleep, specifically stages 3 and 4 (which are medium deep and deep sleep), promote the growth and renewal of bodily tissue, while REM sleep is important for the growth and maintenance of the brain.

Oswald refers to the results of other researchers, who have found that after strenuous physical activity the proportion of the deeper stages of sleep is increased. After great expenditure of energy, the body needs to have its tissues replenished, and apparently the deep-sleep stages offer the best conditions for this. Since thyroid gland hormones, like physical activity, increase the expenditure of energy, it fits well into Oswald's theory that people who suffer from excessive functioning of the thyroid gland and who therefore quickly lose weight, spend an increased proportion of their night's sleep in stages 3 and 4. On the other hand, patients whose thyroid glands are underworking do not achieve stages 3 and 4, but these stages start when the patients are given thyroid gland hormone.

Moreover, children whose bodies are still growing spend more time than adults in deep sleep. Investigations have shown that, specifically in stages 4 and 5, the pituitary gland secretes growth hormone into the blood.

And what is the evidence for REM sleep really playing the rôle in supporting the brain which Oswald ascribes to it? Animals and men have most REM sleep at a time when their brains are most strongly developed. With man this phase comes in the last weeks before birth, and in fact the amount of REM sleep with premature babies is even greater than with ordinary new-born babies. Oswald interprets the continuing increase in REM sleep after narcotic poisoning, for instance, as a sign that brain damage leads to long-lasting repair processes taking place in the brain.

His theory is supported also by an investigation of patients who have had speech disorders caused by brain injuries from accidents. With patients who recovered well after the accident, the researchers observed on average a good deal more REM sleep (twenty per cent of the whole sleeping time) than with patients whose condition did not improve satisfactorily (only 12.7 per cent).

A researcher in Colorado, J. Stoyva, made subjects for a period wear glasses through which they saw everything upside down. Gradually they got used to it. Doubtless an important learning process was bound up with this. It was marked by a big increase in REM sleep.

We are all continually learning, in the sense that our brains are gathering new impressions and assessing experiences. So it seems plausible by Oswald's theory that we also need REM sleep for learning even when the brain is not damaged, not under the influence of psychoactive drugs, and not bewildered by knowledge-hungry scientists with their spectacles conjuring up a topsy-turvy world!

Do dreams help us forget?

Oswald does not offer any explanation for the dreams in REM sleep. Unless we attach no special significance to these strange products of the human mind (which contradicts the impressions dreams often leave behind), they must have some cause. Two British scientists, the psychologist Christopher Evans and the computer expert Edward Arthur Newman of the National Physical Laboratory in Teddington, Middlesex, produced a surprising but perhaps quite plausible theory: the brain forgets through dreams.

Evans and Newman start from experiences with computers. As the memory-stores of these 'electronic brains' need at regular intervals to be cleared of superfluous and outdated information, the brain too throws out ballast—in dreams. The two dream-interpreters argue that the re-programming of computers can only take place when they are out of action. The brain is never out of action, but at least in sleep it is not concerned with its surroundings.

If computers are not regularly cleared of superfluous information, their working speed is reduced and their functioning is impaired. With loss of REM sleep—say Evans and Newman—the brain's efficiency suffers accordingly, so it hastens to make up its losses of dream sleep at the earliest opportunity. The information which the brain wants to clear out is extremely varied, which is why dreams easily become so chaotic: the various parts of the dream 'plot' are often loosely and/or irrationally connected with each other. But normally the sleeper does not have any awareness of what he is dreaming. It is only when he awakens from a dream that he finds out that he has dreamed at all. Our uncertainty over most dreams seems expedient to Evans and Newman because the dream is just what the brain is wanting to clear out. They also have a theory on why the few dreams we remember are often charged with emotion: these are just the dreams most designed to disturb our sleep—and it is only under such conditions that we learn something about our dreams.

If, say the two computer experts, it one day proves possible to build electronic brains which independently check their own programmes against reality, then it could be stated without absurdity that these computers would also dream.

This prospect, however, looks some way in the future; and meanwhile there are many basic questions for sleep researchers to answer, so that theories and hypotheses are replaced by confirmed knowledge.

19

Manipulating Memory

'Want to be intelligent?' asked the *Journal of the American Medical Association*. 'Swallow a professor.' This invitation to cannibalism was the heading to a series of experiments from which in 1962 the psychologist James McConnell at the University of Michigan drew the sensational conclusion that learning is edible.

This was what had happened in the experiments. McConnell had taught flat-worms little tricks, such as contracting on a flash of light. When the worms had mastered their lesson satisfactorily, he reduced them to a pulp, which he then fed to worms of the same species; other worms of that species also became cannibals but on a pulp of untrained worms. When he began training the two groups of cannibals to do the same trick, those which had been fed on trained members of their species learned their task twice as quickly as those fed on the untrained. McConnell, the discoverer of memory transfer, has already recognised the far-reaching possibilities which might result from his experiments at some not too distant time. 'Why should we simply waste a respected professor's whole knowledge which he has accumulated over the years,' he asked in a lecture, 'merely because he has reached the age of retirement?'

After a slight moment of shock, thinking of his trained worms being cut up and set before untrained worms as food, his colleagues realised he was not suggesting a new solution for the geriatric problem. What he wanted was work by the pharmaceutical industry on synthesising molecules of memory which would allow students to absorb through pills the knowledge which at present they have to cram laboriously into their heads.

Since then scientists in many laboratories have transmitted from one creature to another what the involuntary brain supplier had learned beforehand. Whole brigades not only of flat-worms but of goldfish, mice and rats were patiently trained for the single aim of allowing other members of the species to acquire knowledge without effort. One of the memory substances could even be analysed. Once its structure was known, chemists produced it synthetically, and in fact the artificial product was just as good for instilling learning as the natural substance obtained from the brains of trained creatures.

Did the researchers thereby clear up exactly what memory is? Is it nothing more than an assortment of substances in the brain, which have stored various memories according to their different chemical structure? The problem has proved much harder than that. Up to the present day, memory has been one of the brain's functions about which our knowledge is still very scanty—certainly in comparison with the intensive efforts applied by brain researchers to this very problem.

Manipulation does not need complete knowledge of the connections. How memory content is transferred from one brain to another without the usual learning process being brought into action was discovered by scientists before they could agree on what actually happened in the brain when it remembered something. Still, there seems a good chance today that one of the many theories put forward by memory

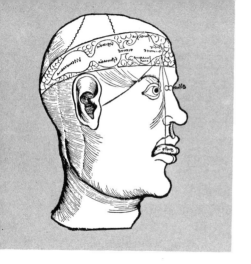

As this picture from 1504 shows, medieval sages believed that the memory was lodged in the posterior of the brain.

researchers, taking into account the results so far achieved, may prove to be correct.

Many kinds of memory

Everyone knows from his own experience how complicated memory is. We usually talk about 'memory' in the singular, and this in itself fails to do justice to the complexity of the phenomena which anybody can easily observe about the storing of information in his own brain. There are different kinds of memory, as most people realise to their cost through the limits of their learning capacity.

Many have remarkable powers of memory for visual impressions, sometimes a total recall of scenes from the past. Others have acoustic impressions 'engraved on their memory' with special vividness. Others again have a particularly good memory for the spoken or written word. They have an easy time of it at school and anywhere that instruction has to be drummed in; yet they may completely lack the capacity for absorbing, say, visual images. Such people may very well remember the name of someone they have met, but forget what he looks like; while with the visually gifted it is the other way round.

Besides different specialities our memory seems to have several 'layers'. Most of what is stored in it we can activate without difficulty, and our brains, in fact, show an amazing capacity for memory when we are having a conversation: the recall of a wide variety of information takes place quite fluently without our needing to strain ourselves in the process.

There are many things, on the other hand, which we can only remember with difficulty. Some just will not come to us, however hard we try; yet we know they are still 'there'. Quite often what we were looking for comes up surprisingly at a moment when we have started thinking of something completely different.

Finally, there is a mass of things which we once knew but which we cannot remember with the best will in the world, however persistently we brood over it. We can no longer describe a picture we once saw, or give a name we once knew. Yet even this apparently forgotten item is not completely wiped out of our brain. If we are shown the picture, we recognise it again; if told the forgotten name, we know it is the right one.

We can also distinguish between short-term and long-term memory. If we look up a number in the telephone directory, our memory takes it in, but forgets it again as soon as we have dialled. Arrangements we have to make, dates we have fixed, and most of the knowledge we hastily soak up the day before an exam, do not as a rule last beyond the short-term memory. A telephone number we often dial, on the other hand, has as good prospects of being fixed in our long-term memory as learning matter often repeated. But again it is not that simple: many things we should like to retain and work hard to remember, just will not go into the long-term memory; yet useless details will sometimes find a lasting place in the brain without our specially attending to them, let alone making an effort to impress them on our memory.

Subjective impressions (which can be deceptive, as was

shown in the last chapter for dreams) would suggest that the line between short-term and long-term memory is not so sharp as the two terms seem to imply. Our experience teaches us that forgetting is not fixed to a particular time. What the brain has taken in can be forgotten after seconds, minutes, hours or days, but also after weeks, months or years. Yet the results of experiments with animals and also observations on patients show that the division into short-term and long-term memory may be justified.

For instance, after concussion, poisoning or electro-convulsive therapy (electric shock treatment) patients often cannot recall events which took place directly before the interference in the brain's normal activity. A period of ten to thirty minutes is blurred, while memories further back are not affected. Serious brain injuries can result in loss of memory going far deeper into the past. It is reassuring and astonishing that as recovery proceeds the memory gradually starts working again. But the memories which have vanished from short-term memory, say after concussion, never return.

On the memory trail

Unless one goes in for mystical conceptions, one is driven to the conclusion that whenever we increase our memory, a real change takes place in the brain, though perhaps only a tiny one. The presumption that mind exists independently of matter stopped this rather obvious idea from gaining any attention till the late nineteenth century. In 1904 the German zoologist Richard Semon put forward the hypothesis that any stimulus an organism receives, any information a living creature has absorbed, leaves behind a characteristic material trace in the nervous system, which he called an 'engram', and to which that creature can reach back as required in later life.

Many researchers set about looking for engrams. The most

extensive investigations were undertaken by the American psychologist Karl S. Lashley. He started from the premise that every engram must be lodged at a particular place in the brain, in fact in the cerebrum, as a trace of any information received in the brain.

He first trained laboratory animals to carry out definite tasks reliably. One task for rats, his favourite subjects, might consist, for instance, in running the only possible way through a maze. When they had learned how to do this, he removed a part of their cerebral cortex, expecting that according to where the part removed was, some rats would have had the knowledge taught them cut away with the brain tissue. In this way he hoped to find out where the information was stored.

His hopes were not fulfilled. Whichever part of the cerebral cortex he destroyed, the rats retained the knowledge acquired. He never managed to discover the location of an engram. How well they could still carry out their task after the operation did not depend on the site of the surgery but only on the amount of cortex removed. With a loss of half, for instance, their performance was still about half as good as before the operation. So what they had learnt seemed to be distributed over the whole cerebral cortex.

The first large-scale attempt to come to grips with memory in the laboratory had failed. In fact, after spending much of his research career on the 'memory trail', Lashley wrote in 1950, when contemplating the results of his work, 'I sometimes feel that the only conclusion to be drawn is: learning is not possible at all.'

But as everyone knows, of course, learning is an everyday phenomenon. So researchers, while they accepted Lashley's disappointing finding that information is not stored in a particular part of the cerebral cortex, did not give up the search for memory traces.

The brain works electrically. Is memory too an electrical activity? This theory was put forward at the beginning of the 'fifties by Eccles. He suggested that information was transmitted by the sense organs to the brain as electrical impulses and then circulated further in the brain. According to this view, reverberatory activity occurs between certain nerve cells, such as can be used in computers for storing information; and the information is available in the brain as memory content so long as the appropriate reverberations continue.

The Göttingen brain researcher Paul Glees tested the theory and refuted it by showing that anything learned was retained even if the brain's electrical functioning was switched off. He cooled down the brains of anaesthetised monkeys to 18–19°C (64–66°F) and thereby wiped out the electrical activity, as the EEG indicated. For three-quarters of an hour, while the brain remained at this temperature, no current was circulating in the brain. But when the monkeys woke after their brains had been warmed again, they had not lost their memory. They carried out tasks for which they had been trained as easily as before the brain-cooling. So electrical reverberations could not be the information-storers which research was looking for.

Finally, at the third attempt, scientists managed to track down changes in the brain connected with the storage of information. The working hypothesis that memory content in the brain could be chemically fixed, that is in the form of particular molecules, proved fruitful. The first molecules tried were the huge ones of nucleic acids, which are made up of relatively few constituents on the box-of-bricks system. Since there are thousands of permutations of these constituents, it means an immense number of possibilities for their arrangement. Could it be that different nucleic acid molecules represented different memory contents?

The idea was supported by the fact that nucleic acids had already been shown to have a memory function, though in a different sense from what one generally understands by memory. The genes in the cell nuclei consist of a group of these acids—the deoxyribonucleic acids (DNA for short). Many different sorts of DNA make up the structural plan of a living creature, which is transmitted from one generation to another. DNA, say the biologists, is the basis of hereditary or species memory. From the DNA, copies are made in the cell nucleus which consist in a second group of nucleic acids, ribonucleic acids (RNA for short). These travel to the cell's protein factories, where they are 'translated' into protein molecules, which then control the metabolic processes in the body. There are also proteins in unimaginable variety, also put together on the box-of-bricks system—though their constituents come out of a different box of bricks from the constituents of the nucleic acids.

The idea arose that RNA molecules—different from those involved in the hereditary process—might also serve as stores for the information which every living creature takes in during its life. Investigation in 1952 had shown with rabbits that, in the nerve cells of the retina (which develops as part of the brain), the RNA content is constantly increasing during the first ten weeks of life, but only when the rabbits are capable of seeing anything. With rabbits brought up in darkness the RNA content of the retina cells remained small.

Although these findings had nothing directly to do with memory, they showed that nerve cells reacted to stimuli with chemical changes. A Swedish researcher, Holger Hydén, at Gothenburg University, came near the core of the problem in the early 'sixties with extensive investigations. He had developed methods, much admired by his colleagues, making it possible to prepare individual nerve cells from the brain tissue and provide a chemical analysis of the tiny structures. He now taught young rats to balance on a wire which went steeply upwards at an angle of forty-five degrees; there was food at the top. Subsequent examination of the tightrope-trained rats showed that in the nerve cells of the balance centre (in the brain stem) the RNA content had considerably increased—compared to rats which had not learnt the tightrope act—and the RNA also had unusual composition.

Cleverness through cannibalism

Meanwhile McConnell in Michigan had for years been concerned with his training of flat-worms. These lower forms of life, seldom more than two or three millimetres long, very common in streams and rivers, ponds and lakes, have only a very primitive nervous system, but still the beginnings of a 'brain', as one may describe the concentration of nerve cells in the front part of the worm. These worms have extraordinary powers of regeneration: if one is cut into fifty pieces, under favourable conditions every piece will grow into a complete new worm.

McConnell had first to tackle the tiresome job of finding out whether these primitive creatures could be taught anything at all. They could. In a plastic trough filled with water, through which he was able to transmit electric current, they learned on a flash of light to contract as violently as they would otherwise only do after an electric shock.

The next question was how far the knowledge of the 'trained' worms would remain if he divided them. He cut them into two halves, waited a month till complete worms had grown up again from the halves, and then tested how much knowledge had lasted. He expected that the worms which had grown from the head halves would still retain their training, but not those from the tail halves, which had been obliged to grow a new head plus brain. But in fact these could perform their act almost as perfectly as the halves which 'started' their new life with brains. Moreover, McConnell reported, 'even when we cut the trained worms into three or four pieces, with the worms newly regenerated from those parts, the perfectly retained learning effects were still shown'.

McConnell with his flat-worms had thus arrived at a similar point to Lashley with his rats: the knowledge acquired could not be localised. But now there was Hydén's theory whereby RNA functioned as memory substance. If certain substances actually served as knowledge stores, McConnell reflected, knowledge must be transferable from one creature to another.

So he made his sensational cannibal experiments. He first tried to transplant pieces of trained worms into untrained ones, without success; then he made the trained worms into food and achieved the hoped-for result. He could also prove that RNA was responsible for the transference of knowledge: in a series of experiments he made an extract, containing the RNA, of the pulp of trained worms, and injected it into the untrained ones. The worms which received the extract learned their task a good deal faster than untreated worms.

His results caused an immense stir in the scientific world. Many researchers found them basically incredible. The scepticism grew when some research teams reported they had had no success at all in training flat-worms. But this discrepancy was cleared up, as the failures proved to have occurred with a particularly stupid kind of flat-worm! The tests were successful when McConnell supplied worms from his own stud. 'Many of us, myself included, were sceptical,' confessed the American William L. Byrne from Durham (U.S.A.). 'But the attempt to refute James McConnell has refuted us instead.'

Goldfish made forgetful

More and more researchers reported results indicating the importance of RNA for the memory. There were continual surprises. Allen Jacobsen at the University of

California in Los Angeles reported that through RNA knowledge could even be transmitted from one animal species to another. He trained hamsters to run to the feeding bowl at a light or sound signal. When they could do this reliably, he extracted the RNA from their brains and injected the extract into rats, who thereupon showed the same reaction as the hamsters had done before.

Other scientists found that proteins also had something to do with the memory. Bernard Agranoff at the University of Michigan taught goldfish, in an aquarium divided by a barrier, to swim over the barrier into the other half directly a light went on. This was the only way they could avoid a painful electric shock.

Directly after their training he injected them beneath the skull with a substance which blocked the forming of protein in the brain—the antibiotic, puromycin; the fish quickly forgot what they had learned. In other experiments, where puromycin was not injected till an hour after the training, there was no effect: what they had learned was fixed in the brain. If it was injected before the training, they first learned as normal, but did not retain the lesson for long; after the training they quickly forgot it all.

The substance inhibiting the forming of protein obviously stopped information being absorbed into the long-term memory, although the short-term memory functioned normally. Ideas about the chemical aspects of the learning process could thus be refined. After the experiments with an inhibiting substance, which also gave positive results on mice, it was accepted that, in learning, special kinds of RNA came up immediately, which then served as sources for the production of specific kinds of protein for the long-term memory.

Transferred fear of the dark

Success was soon achieved also in transmitting knowledge

through proteins, even in identifying one of these and exactly reproducing it in the laboratory. This was done by Georges Ungar at the Baylor University in Houston, Texas. With his artificially produced molecules he transmitted to mice a fear of darkness which he had taught to rats.

Normally both rats and mice prefer darkness to light. If in a laboratory they are left the choice between a dark and a light part of their cage, they spend most of the time in the dark part. Ungar now made them dislike the darkness by giving them an electric shock whenever they tried to slip into the dark part of the cage. They quickly learned to fear the dark.

After the rats had learned this, they were killed. From their brains Ungar and his team prepared an extract which they injected into mice. Before the injection the mice, who never received an electric shock, spent on average 130 to 140 seconds in the dark during a period of 180 seconds. After the injection darkness was suspect to them, although they had had no sort of bad experiences with it. During the test period they spent no more than 50 to 60 seconds in the dark. This striking reduction was not shown by mice injected with a brain extract from untrained rats or from rats trained to other behaviour.

To obtain the fear-of-the-dark substance from the rats' brains in as pure a form as possible, Ungar's team taught over four thousand rats to fear the dark part of the cage. They collected five kilograms of rats' brains trained to fear of the dark. This contained fractions of a milligram of the effective substance; small as the amount was, it was enough to establish the chemical composition. It proved to be a protein, or more exactly a peptide. Like proteins, peptides consist of amino acids which have joined up into chains, but scientists do not call such chains proteins unless at least a hundred amino acids are joined together. The fear-of-the-dark substance is made up of fifteen amino acid constituents which Ungar could identify. He christened the substance scotophobin, from the Greek words for 'dark' and 'fear'.

After the composition of scotophobin was discovered, it could be synthesised. Wolfgang Parr, a colleague of Ungar's in Houston, produced a preparation which had the same effect in the brain of mice as natural scotophobin. It later proved that scotophobin can even make goldfish afraid of a dark area within their aquarium.

'I believe', said Ungar, 'that scotophobin is the first code-word of an incredibly large series. Our experiences are locked up in such codewords and stored in the central nervous system "on recall". Once the laws of a code are known, it can be turned back into the original information. It is there-fore conceivable that with the knowledge of the neural code we should become capable of reading the information locked in the peptides. It would then be possible even to synthesise molecules with all kinds of potential new informa-tion, which could then produce the corresponding be-haviour in the brain.'

Ungar is already working on the identification of other memory substances. He is collecting brains of rats which have been trained to react positively to a noise stimulus. They are normally frightened by noise, and he is experi-menting with a substance which trains goldfish, contrary to their normal preference, to choose a green light rather than a red one.

The goldfish training, carried out with rewards for correct behaviour and without punishments for wrong behaviour, was developed by the Göttingen researchers Hans Peter Zippel and Gotz Domagk at the University's Physiological Institute. They taught the fish to like water made sour by vinegar or bitter by quinine, and by brain extracts trans-ferred the strange preferences in colour and taste to other goldfish which had never received a reward for 'unnaturally' liking a green light or bitter taste. Ungar hopes to train twenty thousand goldfish in order to identify the liking-for-green-substance, which he will then perhaps call chloro-philin. Probably this substance is also a peptide.

It must be admitted that Ungar's work is still very controversial. Many other researchers have not found his results, and even if they did would still claim that a non-memory explanation is possible.

What is learning?

Although today there are many discoveries about memory, we cannot say that they have already led to a clear idea about the way it works. Scientists who hope to build a complete picture from the results of memory research so far, must start from the following premises:

(1) There are no narrowly defined sites for particular memory contents. What we know is distributed, instead, over wide regions of the cerebral cortex.

(2) Memory contents in the long-term memory are not designed in the form of electrical reverberations, whereas it is possible that electrical activity does play a part in short-term memory. Brain currents are certainly involved, as studies on EEGs show, in the activation of stored knowledge.

(3) For the functioning of long-term memory (so that it can take in information from short-term memory, or, according to another theory, so that information can be recalled from long-term memory) there is an important mechanism which can be put out of action by interference with the hippocampus, part of the limbic system (see Chapter 8).

(4) During the learning process substances grow up through which the knowledge acquired can be transmitted from one brain to another. These are RNA and peptides, two very variable classes of substances.

The memory researchers were surprised at first that they found not just one class of memory molecules but two.

However, since in genetic research, looking for species memory, close relations had been discovered between RNA and proteins, the surprise did not last long. The general view today is that, in learning, RNA molecules are the first to be formed, and that it is their function to produce proteins or peptides which are the 'executive' molecules for the functioning of memory.

It may now be asked: where does the RNA come from; and what exactly do the peptides do in the brain?

The first question has not yet been fully answered, though it raises others with far-reaching philosophical consequences. We know that RNA molecules, which are active in the hereditary process, are formed as copies of DNA molecules. Are memory RNA molecules formed in a similar way, according to the pattern of DNA molecules, the only difference being that this occurs on an impulse which must be connected with the receiving of information in the brain? This would mean that any living creature can learn only within a framework determined by hereditary factors.

This idea is confirmed in practice if the learning capacities of different animal species are compared to each other: limits of capacity depending on the species are clearly recognisable. But when we look at human learning, the situation becomes more complicated. Our brain today takes in information which certainly was not presented to the brains of our ancestors. Our society and our environment are not the same as those of our ancestors. We can probably assume that our brains today learn more than the brains of people alive earlier; but even without this assumption, the differences in the character of the information learned are unmistakable.

It is hard to imagine that these qualitative differences should have no significance at all for the basic processes of memory storage and recall. Is the development of man's culture and civilisation, which leads to different memory contents being imprinted on brains from generation to generation, only a single theme with variations? Does it need no new memory substances? If not, we have to explain how one and the same substance can store and activate different memory contents.

'Learning consists in remembering information which has already lodged for generations in man's soul.' Such was the teaching, nearly two thousand five hundred years ago, of Socrates, who knew nothing of DNA, RNA and proteins and who had no inkling of the importance of the brain. The opposite point of view is represented by the seventeenth-century English philosopher John Locke, who said that learning is based on experience. He compared a man's memory at birth with an unhewn block of white marble: as the stonemason carves letters into the marble, so life stamps experience into the memory.

Who would dispute that learning is based on experience? Yet it is established today that man is not born with an empty brain. Even before birth, without having gathered any experience, the brain can co-ordinate some things, for instance sucking movements. Above all, it has been shown that a child goes through the separate stages in growing up according to a strict timetable. What he can learn at different ages is fixed in his genes.

The block of marble, to keep Locke's analogy, although practically unhewn, has marks showing what can and what cannot be carved into it. We can scarcely assume that such indications would include formulae from nuclear physics, modern painting or specific unforgettable experiences. So we have yet to find out a mean between the two extremes suggested by Socrates and Locke, as to what learning is and how it is to be explained.

If we now tackle the second question, on the action in the brain of the peptides as memory molecules, we quickly reach the shaky ground of unconfirmed theories. It seems certain that the peptide molecules do not represent magnetic tapes from which the memory contents can be played as required. 'This is biological nonsense,' declared Holger Hydén, with the agreement of most memory researchers.

When we recall that the brain consists of a network of nerve cells with incredibly complex connections, the question arises: what function can the memory peptides have in this jungle of electrical 'wiring'? Till today the possibility cannot be excluded that the body of glia cells between the nerve cells (ten times more of them than there are nerve cells), or even the spaces without cells which occupy one fifth of the brain, are of decisive importance for the memory.

One of the many theories for interpreting what happens in memory from the experimental findings has been put forward by Ungar. This hypothesis is that when a human baby is born, it already has all the nerve cells but not all the connections between them: learning therefore consists in new connections being formed between the nerve cells. So that the new paths for nerve signals can be opened up, the peptides noted as memory substances are needed, with each kind of peptide responsible for a large number of connections. Ungar believes that in the brains of laboratory animals taught by him to fear the dark, some hundred thousand to a million new connections have been created by scotophobin. In his view ten million peptides would be enough to fix the information lodged in the brain of a human adult.

Ungar recognises himself how far his theory is, like many other hypotheses, from offering a satisfactory explanation for memory. He admits it is amazing that such a system could be responsible for the incredible complexity of the human memory. How could one explain, for example, in molecular terms, the way we remember a poem, a philosophic doctrine or a scientific theory?

Injections of learning?

Although we do not understand the connections, it is quite possible that memory substances will soon be found for use on human brains as well. We can imagine, say, that many behavioural disorders, at present very hard to treat, may be corrected by learning substances.

There are the unfortunate people who suffer from phobias and compulsion neuroses. Some, for instance, feel faint at the mere idea of going out of doors; they have a fear of open spaces which is called agoraphobia. Others are panic-stricken if left in the dark—like Ungar's rats and mice. Others have a morbid fear of uncleanness or infection, which makes them keep washing continually (the Lady Macbeth syndrome, it might be called); they feel this need after every contact with another person or a much used object like a door-handle. They cannot stop performing actions which they know to be completely irrational; indeed compulsion neuroses and phobias bear no relation to the intelligence of those affected. Sometimes a long course of psychotherapy helps, but often all the efforts to help are in vain.

Might not appropriate learning substances remove the disorders? Through such substances the agoraphobes could come to like open spaces, and the 'scotophobes' enjoy the dark. The prospects for this do not appear too slim, now that the fear-of-the-dark learning substance has possibly been isolated, analysed and synthesised. It is especially important in this connection that a single substance can produce the same effect with different animal species. Other learning substances modifying behaviour, which are identified in tests on animals, may therefore be found to work with men also and so be of use as models for the synthetic production of healing psychoactive drugs.

Alcoholics, after a 'drying out' course, are all too likely to relapse; perhaps they might be cured by a fear-of-alcohol substance which stops the addiction. One learning substance might free people from their compulsion to be always washing, with other such substances arousing more cheerful interests. One can think of any number of possibilities for the beneficial use of learning substances.

In the longer view all mankind should be able to profit by them. 'One day,' wrote the worm-researcher McConnell, 'it might become possible to provide certain kinds of knowledge directly, the somatic way, that is through incorporation of the appropriate "memory molecules".' Before venturing on this prognosis, however, he wisely gave the warning: 'Let me pursue my speculation to its furthest limit, which at present will doubtless seem quite incredible.'

Only a few years after these remarks, the idea that learning substances may replace laborious cramming does not appear quite so incredible; but there are still considerable difficulties to be overcome. It would be wrong, therefore, to arouse exaggerated hopes. Learning substances will not make schools and universities superfluous all that soon. A packet of pills labelled 'Chinese for beginners' or drops enabling everyone to understand without effort what is really meant by the theory of relativity—such attractive novelties are not yet in sight.

With man, in contrast to flat-worms, RNA and peptides are affected by the digestive process; but that is not the only thing which stands in the way of our quickly dispensing with traditional educational methods. This obstacle could be avoided by having memory molecules injected. It seems a more serious handicap that our knowledge about the complex processes involved, say, in learning a language, is still extremely limited. It is possible, however, that here again manipulations may become possible before the laws they follow have been grasped in detail.

Certainly the dangers of an abuse of learning substances are great. Autocrats have always tried to influence their subjects' brains. Memory substances would make it easier and perhaps ensure a hundred per cent success rate. Ungar is 'of course aware of the possibility of misuse of these discoveries. This problem, however, is raised with every scientific advance—and the only possible answer, I am convinced, is to communicate the discoveries to the public.'

What will the public do with the discoveries when it has them? Obviously it will ask whether the advantages for humanity which may be expected from the chemical transfer of memory contents outweigh the risk of dangerous manipulations. This risk applies to almost all fields of modern brain research, so how is brain research to proceed at all? Should brain researchers be allowed to continue independently as they have done till now, in the hope that all will be for the best, or should efforts be made to put the brakes on?

20

Apollo Programme for Brain Research

Besides allowing brain researchers their head unsupervised and putting the brakes on their work, there is a third possibility: to make brain research the focal point of future scientific planning. This, I believe, is not only the right line but the line which must be taken.

Though with due criticism, and checks on the successes achieved, governments should give the most generous and whole-hearted sponsorship to all brain research projects which appear practical, if necessary at the cost of plans in other research fields. I consider it justifiable to declare brain research international priority number one.

For today the most important thing of all must surely be to solve what Sir John Eccles called 'the elemental problem with which man finds himself confronted'.

In view of its significance for every single human being, it is remarkable how little we know about the brain. Well might Ungar deplore the gaping abyss between our immense knowledge of the physical universe and our almost complete ignorance of the way our minds work. The consequences of such ignorance are grave.

Doctors are agreed today that the brain plays a considerable part in the development of many widespread diseases, not only mental and nervous ones. Many which the patients think have a purely physical cause come into the large group of psychosomatic illnesses. Authorities estimate that twenty per cent of all the patients visiting a general practitioner or specialist for internal complaints complain of troubles in which psychological factors play a decisive part. The list of complaints which may be psychosomatically caused is long. It includes diseases of the heart and circulation, of the stomach and intestines; compulsive eating and anorexia (loss of appetite), chronic headaches and migraines, breathing disorders, skin diseases, various women's diseases, impotence, etc., etc. There are also the many patients who complain of various troubles, without the doctors' being able to find evidence of organic disorders. But of course abdominal and duodenal ulcers, asthma attacks and dangerous rises in blood pressure can be equally psychosomatic.

For all these complaints doctors repeatedly prescribe drugs, sometimes undertake surgery, offer advice on how to lead a healthy life, carry out psychotherapy. The successes, if any, are short-lived. The logic seems clear: we know too little about the human brain; too little about the causes of the reactions in the body which make many people ill; too little about the posibilities of providing a lasting cure for these sick people.

But even those who are not sick are often in difficulties because of their own brains and the brains of others. Living together in any human society is rich in conflicts, most of which on calm reflection are both completely superfluous and do more harm than good to all concerned. Both individually and socially, we are all victims of unharmonious brain development.

Endowed with reason and the capacity for logical thinking, we also have to live with mechanisms in our brain which can at any time suppress all the arguments of reason. Worse still, these powerful mechanisms from earlier stages of brain development contrive to make use of reason in the most irrational way. To develop weapons, to organise wars and acts of terrorism demands very considerable logical thinking; yet such undertakings are extremely irrational. Indeed, we can easily recognise the full extent of the irrationality of others, especially when their quarrel is no concern of ours. But we are often helpless against our own irrationality, even to the point of self-destruction if we are unlucky.

Nothing in man's history indicates that things have taken a turn for the better over all these centuries. Philosophers have brooded in vain, moralists and religious leaders have prophesied and preached in vain, reformers have tried in vain to design or produce new forms of society. One immense, untested hope remains; the most thorough and purposeful exploration of the brain. Science has now reached a stage when it has prospects of fathoming more successfully the contradictions as well as the wonders of the centre of human life.

But what of the menace of dangerous manipulations? Certainly the possibilities of manipulation grow with the increase of knowledge. But how serious are the dangers which may result from brain research—compared to the present horrors of this world? When I was working on the end of this book, the war in Vietnam had reached a new peak; Protestant and Catholic fanatics were fighting each other in Northern Ireland; in Turkey and the Argentine revolutionaries who considered themselves humanitarians had kidnapped people completely uninvolved in their conflicts and murdered them after attempts at blackmail against hated regimes had failed.

I mention these four countries particularly, to show that the horror goes all round the world. Peace reigns between the two great powers whose quarrel could lead to the destruction of all human civilisation. But this peace is little more than the absence of direct armed conflict. The relationship is not determined by constructive co-operation but by mutual suspicion and pinpricks—however the pricks can be applied without great risk. The basis of this peace is simply a balance of destructive power, a balance which can be disturbed at any time.

How much does mankind risk if it gives priority to brain research? My belief is that although it has some things to lose, it has far more to gain. Of course the risk which brain research brings with it should be kept to a minimum; and, as has been stressed throughout this book, the greater our vigilance, the smaller the risk will be. The 'Apollo' brain research programme should certainly include massive public education through the press and all other media on the potential benefits as well as the inevitable dangers. At least in the Western democracies, where far the largest amount of brain research is carried out, a variety of opinions and a control through a wide spectrum of publications are assured. In these circumstances governments and scientific departments should not find it easy to misuse the results of research secretly for dubious forms of manipulation.

We are pretty well at the beginning of the adventure of brain research, and basic work on a broad front is still needed. But beyond that we should formulate the objectives of such research. The initiators of America's Project Apollo had set themselves the aim of putting the first men on the moon; this was an impressive example of purposeful research planning. That the aim of their expensive and intensive efforts was insignificant by comparison, does not diminish the organisational achievement. The experience gained from this planned research success might help greatly towards the focal point in a brain research programme.

As priority aim for this programme, I propose an 'all-out attack' on human violence. Brain researchers have already made the first discoveries about the mechanisms which cause violence; and brain manipulation to suppress it would be likely to win public approval. Even partial success would considerably reduce the dangers of such accompanying phenomena as hunger for power and ideological fanaticism. Doubtless there would be many political problems involved, but if a 'pacifying' substance were discovered and thoroughly tested, there would surely be ways of using it to 'defuse' many at present insoluble conflicts and to prevent a vast amount of suffering. A substance of this kind does not so far exist; but then nor do any other reliable measures against violent behaviour for large-scale application. We should urgently demand that such a substance be developed.

BIBLIOGRAPHY

Agranoff, Bernard W., *Memory and Protein Synthesis. Scientific American*, June 1967, P. 115–122.

Akert, Konrad, *Struktur und Ultrastruktur von Nervenzellen und Synapsen. Klinische Wochenschrift* 49/1971, P. 509–519.

Alexander, F. G., and S. T. Selesnick, *Geschichte der Psychiatrie.* Konstanz 1969.

Andreoli, Armando, *Zur geschichtlichen Entwicklung der Neuronentheorie.* Basle/Stuttgart 1961.

Apfelbach, R., *Aggressionsforschung durch elektrische Hirnreizung. Umschau,* 5/1971, P. 170–172.

Baker, Peter F., *The Nerve Axon. Scientific American,* March 1966, P. 74–82.

Baust, Walter (Editor), *Ermüdung, Schlaf und Traum,* Frankfurt 1971.

Bay, E., *Sprache, Denken und Gehirn. Umschau,* 10/1963, P. 301–304.

Benzinger, Theodor, *Der Thermostat im Menschen. Bild der Wissenschaft,* 3/1964, P. 50–59 and 3/1965, P. 232–240.

Birkmayer, W., and E. Neumeyer, *Neue Vorstellungen über die biochemischen Ursachen der Depression. Therapeutische Berichte,* 3/1969, P. 147–152.

Blinkov, Samuel M., and Ilja J. Glezer, *Das Zentralnervensystem in Zahlen und Tabellen.* Jena 1968.

Blomquist, A. J., and D. D. Gilboe, *Auditory and Somatic Sensory Responses Evoked in the Cerebral Cortex of the Isolated Dog Brain. Nature*, Vol. 227/1970, P. 409.

Busch, Eduard, *Psychosurgery.* Handbuch der Neurochirurgie, Vol. 6 (1957).

Bushe, Karl-August, and Paul Glees, *Chirurgie des Gehirns und Rückenmarks im Kindes- und Jugendalter.* Stuttgart 1968.

Calder, Nigel, *The Mind of Man.* British Broadcasting Corporation 1970; New York 1971.

Chedd, Graham, *Brain and brawn in a glass dish. New Scientist,* 8. 10. 1970, P. 70–71.

Delgado, José M. R., *Die experimentelle Hirnforschung und die Verhaltensweise. Endeavour,* 69 (1967), P. 149–154.

Diepgen, Paul, *Geschichte der Medizin,* Berlin 1949 (Vol. I), 1951 (Vol. II, First Half) and 1955 (Vol. II, Second Half).

Domagk, G. F., and H. P. Zippel, *Biochemie der Gedächtnisspeicherung. Naturwissenschaften,* 4/1970, P. 152–162.

Eccles, John, *Funktionsweisen des neuralen Mechanismus im Zentralnervensystem. Naturwissenschaftliche Rundschau,* 4/1967, P. 139–151.

Eccles, John, and Donald MacKay, *The challenge of the brain. Science Journal,* April 1967, P. 79–83.

Euler, U. S. von, *Synthese, Speicherung und Freisetzung des adrenergischen Neurotransmitters. Klinische Wochenschrift,* 9/1971, P. 524.

Evans, Christopher, *The Stuff of Dreams. New Scientist,* 18. 5. 1967, P. 409–410.

Evans, Christopher, and E. A. Newman, *Dreaming: an analogy from computers. New Scientist,* 26. 11. 1964, P. 577–579.

Fallaci, Oriana, *The dead body & the living brain. Look,* 24/1967, P. 99–114.

Farber, Seymour M., and Roger H. L. Wilson, *Control of the Mind,* New York 1961.

Fisher, Alan E., *Chemical Stimulation of the Brain. Scientific American,* June 1964, P. 60–68.

Freeman, Walter, and James W. Watts, *Psychochirurgie*, Stuttgart 1949.

Gazzaniga, Michael S., *The Split Brain in Man. Scientific American*, Aug. 1967, P. 24–35.

Gillie, Oliver, *Drug addiction—facts and folklore. Science Journal*, Dec. 1969, P. 75–80.

Glees, Paul, *Meilensteine in der geschichtlichen Entwicklung der Großhirnhistologie*; in: Rothschuh, K. E., *Von Boerhaave bis Berger*, Stuttgart 1964.

Glees, Paul, *Das menschliche Gehirn*, Stuttgart 1968.

Glees, Paul, and Jochen Eschner, *Ist das Gedächtnis strukturell deponiert? Umschau*, 14/1962, P. 435–438.

Gray, E. G., *The Synapse. Science Journal*, May 1967, P. 66–72.

Gregory, Richard L., *Auge und Gehirn. Zur Psychophysiologie des Sehens*, Munich 1966.

Grossman, Sebastian P., *Exploring the brain with chemicals. Discovery*, May 1966, P. 19–23.

Grünewald, Helmut, *Schaltplan des Geistes*, Reinbek 1971.

Grünthal, Ernst, *Psyche und Nervensystem*, Berlin 1969.

Hassler, Rolf, *Funktionelle Neuroanatomie und Psychiatrie. Psychiatrie der Gegenwart*, Vol. I/A (1967), P. 173.

Heimann, Hans, *Psychochirurgie. Psychiatrie der Gegenwart*, Vol. I/2 (1963).

Hesse, Erich, *Rausch-, Schlaf- und Genußgifte*, 4th Edition, Stuttgart 1971.

Hitzig, Eduard, *Physiologie und klinische Untersuchungen über das Gehirn*, Berlin 1904.

Hydén, H., *Experiments on learning and memory*, Manuscript May 1968.

Idris, Ildar, *Neues Fach mit großen Ambitionen: Neurosciences. Selecta*, 5/1969, P. 347–352.

Idris, Ildar, *Ein Groß-Computer im ZNS. Selecta*, 40/1969, P. 3203–3209.

Idris, Ildar, *Drogenkult—zwischen Toleranz und Besorgnis. Selecta*, 18/1971, P. 1570–1576.

Jacobsen, A. L., *Chemical transfer of learning. Discovery—*

February 1966.

Janzen, Rudolf, *Elemente der Neurologie auf der Grundlage von Physiologie und Klinik*, Berlin 1969.

Jatzkewitz, Horst, *Biochemische Aspekte in der Psychiatrie.* Umschau, 9/1969, P. 266–270.

Jouvet, Michel, *The States of Sleep. Scientific American*, Feb. 1967, P. 62–72.

Jouvet, Michel, *Biogenic Amines and the States of Sleep. Science*, 3. Jan. 1969, P. 32–40.

Jovanović, Uroš J., *Normal Sleep in Man*, Stuttgart 1971.

Jung, Richard, *Neurophysiologie und Psychiatrie. Psychiatrie der Gegenwart*, Vol. I/1A (1967).

Kandel, Eric R., *Nerve Cells and Behavior. Scientific American*, July 1970, P. 57–70.

Krnjević, K., *Synaptic Transmission in the Brain. Klinische Wochenschrift*, 9/1971, P. 519.

Kulp, Martin, *Menschliches und maschinelles Denken*, Göttingen 1968.

Leineweber, Bernd, *Ein Kopf auf falschem Rumpf. Deutsches Ärzteblatt* 1/1969, P. 50–51.

Löbsack, Theo, *Die unheimlichen Möglichkeiten oder Die manipulierte Seele.* Düsseldorf 1967.

Luria, Alexander Romanovitch, *Traumatic Aphasia, its Syndromes, Psychology and Treatment*, The Hague—Paris 1970.

Luria, Alexander Romanovitch, *The Functional Organization of the Brain. Scientific American*, March 1970, P. 66–78.

MacKay, Donald, *The human brain. Science Journal*, May 1967, P. 43–47.

Matussek, Norbert, *Hirnamine und psychotrope Pharmaka. Umschau*, 12/1966, P. 400–405.

Matussek, Norbert, *Biochemische Aspekte der endogenen Depression. Mitteilungen der Max-Planck-Gesellschaft*, 5/1970, P. 319–331.

McConnell, James V., *Die Suche nach dem Engramm. n + m*, 9/1965, P. 14–26.

Merrem, Georg, *Lehrbuch der Neurochirurgie*, 2nd Edition, Berlin 1964.

Meyer, H.-H., *Arzneimittel gegen seelische Störungen. Deutsche Apotheker-Zeitung*, 30/1967, P. 1041–1044.

Miller, Neal E., *Chemische Reizungen im Gehirn lösen spezifisches Verhalten aus. Umschau*, 8/1966, P. 241–244 and 9/1966, P. 293–294.

Mühr, Alfred, *Das Wunder Menschenhirn*, Olten and Freiburg/Br. 1957.

Netter, Frank H., *The Ciba Collection of Medical Illustrations*, Vol. I. Nervous System.

New Scientist, Brain in a bottle. 28. 11. 1963, P. 525.

New Scientist, Cooling and reviving the brain. 7. 4. 1966, P. 31.

New Scientist, Dream theory receives support. 17. 7. 1969, P. 110.

New Scientist, A chemical control of killing. 19. 2. 1970, P. 342.

New Scientist, RNA may be needed to 'fix' a memory. 12. 3. 1970, P. 495.

New Scientist, Why your brain is so switched on. 22. 7. 1971, P. 180.

New Scientist, Now Scotophobin turns fishy. 13. 1. 1972, P. 64.

Noll, Bernhard W., *Der Massenwahn in Geschichte und Gegenwart. Selecta*, 30/1965, P. 1260–1265.

Olds, James, *Emotional centres in the brain. Science Journal*, May 1967, P. 87–92.

Oswald, Ian, *Sleep, the great restorer. New Scientist*, 23. 4. 1970, P. 170–172.

Ploog, Detlev, *Verhaltensforschung und Psychiatrie. Psychiatrie der Gegenwart*, Vol. I/1B (1964), P. 368–375.

Poeck, K., *Das Limbische System. Deutsche Medizinische Wochenschrift*, 3/1965, P. 131–135.

Poeck, K., *Hat der Mensch zwei Gehirne? Deutsche Medizinische Wochenschrift*, 4/1968, P. 185–187.

Poeck, K., *Die funktionelle Asymmetrie der beiden Hirnhemisphären. Deutsche Medizinische Wochenschrift*, 47/1968, P. 2282–2287.

Poeck, K., *Neurophysiologische Grundlagen der Affektivität. Umschau*, 2/1970, P. 33–36.

Pollak, K., *Wissen und Weisheit der alten Ärzte*, Düsseldorf 1968.

274   BIBLIOGRAPHY

Pollak, Kurt, *Die Heilkunde der Antike*, Düsseldorf 1969.

Portmann, Adolf, *Welche Tiere besitzen die differenziertesten Gehirne?* Umschau, 18/1963, P. 563–566.

Pribram, Karl H., *The Neurophysiology of Remembering.* Scientific American, Jan. 1969, P. 73–86.

Rensch, Bernhard, *Die stammesgeschichtliche Entwicklung der Hirnleistungen. n + m*, 32 (1970), P. 23–31.

Rode, Christian Peter, *Moderne Antidepressiva—Diagnostische Überlegungen und biochemische Aspekte. Deutsche Apotheker-Zeitung*, 1/1972.

Roffwarg, Howard P., Joseph N. Muzio and William C. Dement, *Die ontogenetische Entwicklung des Schlaf-Traumzyklus beim Menschen. Naturwissenschaftliche Rundschau*, 9/1967, P. 363–377.

Rothschuh, K. E., *Physiologie im Werden. Medizin in Geschichte und Kultur*, Vol. 9. Stuttgart 1969.

Sarkissow, S. A., *Grundriß der Struktur und Funktion des Gehirns*, Berlin 1967.

Schadé, J. P., *Einführung in die Neurologie*, Stuttgart 1970.

Schadé, J. P., *Die Funktion des Nervensystems*, Stuttgart 1971.

Scheid, Werner, *Lehrbuch der Neurologie*, 3rd Edition, Stuttgart 1968.

Schipperges, Heinrich, *Die Entwicklung der Hirnchirurgie. Ciba-Zeitschrift* 57, Vol. 7 (1955).

Schlote, Wolfgang, *Struktur und Leistung am Beispiel der Nervenzelle. n + m*, 26 (1969), P. 38–54.

Schmidbauer, Wolfgang, *Es gibt viele künstliche Paradiese. Selecta*, 9/1968, P. 644–656.

Schmidbauer, Wolfgang, and Jürgen vom Scheidt, *Handbuch der Rauschdrogen*, Munich 1971.

Seeds, Nicholas, *Reassembling the brain. New Scientist*, 6. 4. 1972, P. 12–14.

Selecta, Lernen, Erinnern, Gedächtnishemmungen, Speichertheorie. 41/1969, P. 3291–3297.

Selecta, Biochemische und physiologische Aspekte. 42/1969, P. 3344–3350.

Smirnov, Vladimir, *Neuropsychologische Forschungen am Thalamus. Ideen des exakten Wissens*, 4/1969, P. 235–240.

Snider, Ray S., *The Cerebellum. Scientific American*, Aug. 1958, P. 84–90.

Sperry, R. W., *The Growth of Nerve Circuits. Scientific American*, Nov. 1959, P. 68–75.

Sperry, R. W., *The Great Cerebral Commissure. Scientific American*, Jan. 1964, P. 42–52.

Srinivasan, Vasanta, *Where nerve meets nerve. New Scientist*, 22. 10. 1970, P. 187.

Stämpfli, Robert, *Die Erregungsleitung im Nerven. Bild der Wissenschaft*, May 1965, P. 357–367.

Stämpfli, Robert, *Der Erregungsvorgang und seine Fortleitung. Klinische Wochenschrift*, 14/1971, P. 777.

Suda, I., K. Kito and C. Adachi, *Viability of long term frozen cat brain in vitro. Nature*, Vol. 212 (1966), P. 268.

Thomas, Klaus, *Die künstlich gesteuerte Seele*, Stuttgart 1970.

Tritthart, Helmut, *Gedächtnisforschung. Naturwissenschaftliche Rundschau*, 7/1971, P. 289–293.

Ungar, Georges, *Das Gedächtnis in biochemischer Sicht. Umschau*, 6/1971, P. 588–592.

Vernon, Jack, *Inside the Black Room*, New York 1964.

Vernon, Jack, *Sensory deprivation. Science Journal*, Feb. 1966, P. 57–61.

Vogt, Hans-Heinrich, *Reiz—Impuls—Gedanke*, Kosmos-Bibliothek, Vol. 247 (1965).

Wada, Juhn A., Presentation at Nineteenth International Congress of Neurology, New York, 1969.

Walter, W. Grey, *Das lebende Gehirn*, Cologne 1961.

Watermann, Rembert, *Cerebrale Impressionen aus Ägypten. Die Waage*, 3/1963.

Watt, James A. G., *The biochemistry of schizophrenia. New Scientist*, 10. 12. 1970, P. 458–459.

Wechsler, Wolfgang, *Hirnforschung und Elektronenmikroskopie. Mitteilungen der Max-Planck-Gesellschaft*, 3/1963.

White, Robert J., *Isolating the brain. Discovery*, 3/1965, P.

34–37.

White, Robert J., *Das isolierte Gehirn. n + m,* 17 (1967), P. 32–38.

White, Robert J., Maurice S. Albin, George E. Locke and Eugene Davidson, *Brain Transplantation: Prolonged Survival of Brain after Carotid-Jugular Interposition. Science,* Vol. 150 (1965), P. 779–781.

White, Robert J., Maurice S. Albin and Javier Verdura, *Isolation of the Monkey Brain: In vitro Preparation and Maintenance. Science,* Vol. 141 (1963), P. 1060–1061.

Whitteridge, D., *Nerve and brain. New Scientist,* 8. 7. 1965, P. 97–101.

Willows, A. O. D., *Giant Brain Cells in Mollusks. Scientific American, Feb.* 1971, P. 69–75.

Winterstein, H., *Schlaf und Traum,* 2nd Edition, Berlin 1953.

Wooldridge, Dean E., *Machinery of the Brain,* New York 1963.

Young, J. Z., *A Model of the Brain.* Oxford 1964.

Zippel, H. P., and G. F. Domagk, *Versuche zur chemischen Übertragbarkeit erworbener Informationen.* Personal communication to author 1972.

INDEX

acetyl-salicylic acid (aspirin), 136–7
acetylcholine, 125–7, 175, 180, 182
acetylcholine-esterase, 175
acoustic nerve, 201–2
action potential, 164–8, 171–3
Adachi, C., 19
addiction, 131, 134–40, 143–4, 146–50
adrenal cortex, 106
Adrian, E. D., 163
aggression, aggressiveness, 89, 110, 115–7, 122, 127–8
agoraphobia, 261
Agranoff, B., 254
Akert, K., 156
Alcmaeon of Croton, 28
alcohol, alcoholism, etc., 88, 130–2, 135, 140, 145, 148–51, 239, 261
Almeida, L., 86–7
amino acids, 178, 255
aminophenazon (pyramidon), 136
amphetamines, 136–40, 145, 181–2
amphibians, 54
amygdala, 115
analeptics, 141–2, 144, 181
Andersson, B., 123
animal electricity, 161–3
anti-depressants, 131, 142–3, 145, 177–81
Apfelbach, R., 120

aphasia, 74–80
appetite-inhibitors, 138
arachnoid, 35
Aristotle, 29, 226
Aserinsky, E., 228
Asimov, I., 52
aspirin, 136–7
Attardi, D., 193
auditory cortex, 73, 79–81
aversion centres, 99–100, 119
Axelrod, J., 163, 176

barbiturates, 137, 140, 239
basket cells, 208–10
Bay, E., 77–8
Bechterev, V., 89
beetles, 53
Bell, H., 148
belladonna, 133, 145
Berger, H., 230
birds, 231
blindness, cortical, 72
Blomquist, A. J., 16–7
blood-brain-barrier, 178, 235
brain maps, 65–9, 81
brain stem, 8, 32, 34–5, 54, 73, 79, 96, 101–5, 109–10, 204, 206, 231–4
brain stimulation, chemical, 11, 122–8, 213
brain stimulation, electrical, 11, 16–7, 59–61, 69–70, 83–4, 94–100, 105, 107–10, 114–22,

152–3, 213, 232
brain transplants, 20–5
brain ventricles, 31–2, 35
brain-washing, 213, 216–24, 236
breathing centre, 102
Broca, P., 64–5, 74, 76–7
Brodmann, K., 68
bull-frogs, 236
Byrne, W., 253

cactus decoction, 130
caffein, 132, 145, 181
Calder, N., 120–1
cannibal experiments, 244–5,
    252–7
carbachol, 127
cats, 19–20, 38–40, 54, 56, 83,
    95–7, 99, 116, 119–20, 125–6,
    231–4, 238–9
cell bodies, 155–8, 170, 184, 192
cell cultures, 198–200
cerebellum, 8, 32, 34–5, 54, 57,
    79, 101–2, 204–7, 232
cerebrum, 8, 16–7, 32, 34–5, 37,
    54, 57, 62–4, 66–8, 83, 96,
    101–3, 107, 109–10, 202, 204–7,
    209–19, 230, 232–3, 249
chicken embryos, 198–9
chimpanzees, 55, 57, 83, 85–6, 120
chlorophenylalanine, 235
chlorpromazine, 141
chromosomes, 198
Clemente, C. D., 116
climbing fibres, 207, 209–10
coca, 130, 135–6
cocaine, 135–6, 140, 145, 150, 181
cocks, 100
coelenterates, 52
coffee, 130–2, 138–9, 145, 181
cola tree, 132
Columbus, 130
compulsion neuroses, 89, 118,
    261–2
computers, 202–4, 210, 242–3, 250
concussion, 248
consciousness, 210–11
corpus callosum, 34–5, 37–41, 102

cortical homunculus, 68, 70, 209
Coury, J. N., 125
crabs, 53, 195
crocodiles, 112, 236
cytoarchitectonics, 66

Dahl, R., 24
Dale, H. M., 163
deafness, cortical, 73
Deiters, O., 154–5
Delay, J., 141, 144–5
Delgado, J., 70, 94, 100, 115–6,
    118–9, 120–1
Dement, W., 228–9, 231, 238
Demichov, V. P., 21
Democritus, 29
dendrites, 155–60, 170, 172, 184,
    202, 208–9, 226
depressions, 89, 118, 131, 142–3,
    178–80, 234
Descartes, 56, 93
diencephalon, 34–5, 54, 57, 96,
    101, 104, 109–10, 204
dihydroxyphenylalanine, 235
dinosaurs, 54
DNA deoxyribonucleic acids, 251,
    258–9
dogs, 14, 16–7, 21–2, 65, 78, 83,
    99, 189
dolphins, 57–8, 99
Domagk, G., 256
doves, 63–4
dreams, 225–43
Du Bois-Reymond, E., 163
dura mater, 35

eating (feeding) centres, 96
Eccles, J., 9–11, 120, 163, 204–5,
    209–11, 250, 264
Economo, C. v., 68
education, 49–50, 213–4
Edwin Smith Papyrus, 27
Egas Moniz, A. C. de, 86–8, 95
Ehrenberg, C. G., 154
electric shock treatment, 248
electroencephalograph (EEG), 14,
    16, 19, 230–1, 237–8, 250, 257

elephants, 56–7, 158
engrams, 248
enzymes, 179, 181
epileptic fits, 38, 40–1, 59, 79, 110
Erisistratos, 29–30
Erlanger, J., 163
Ervin, F. R., 117
ether, 143–4
Euler, U. v., 163, 176
Evans, C., 242–3

Fallaci, O., 23, 25
fear, 95–6, 99, 105, 110, 136
fear-of-the-dark substance
   (scotophobin), 255–7, 260–1
feedback, 188, 209
filmstrip experiences, 59–61,
   78–81
Fischbach, G., 198–9
fishes, 112, 194, 196
Fisher, A. E., 123–5
flat-worms, 52–3, 244–5, 252–3,
   262
Flourens, M. J. P., 63–4
fly agaric, 133, 182
fore-brain, 54, 85–7, 90, 92–3
Freud, S., 135–6, 226–7
Fritsch, G. T., 65, 83
frogs, 190–4, 196
frontal lobe, 61, 81–5, 93
fuse principle, 164, 168

Gage, Phineas, 82–4, 92
Galen, 30–3, 36
Gall, F. J., 61–5
Galvani, L., 161–2
gamma-amino-butyric acid, 175
Gasser, H. S., 163
Gazzaniga, M. S., 41–4, 46–7, 49
genes, 197–8, 250–1, 258–9
gibbons, 120
Gilboe, D. D., 16–7
giraffes, 158
Glees, P., 26, 250
glia cells, 159–60, 260
glucagon, 125
glutamic acid, 175

glycin, 175
goats, 123
goldfish, 99, 193–4, 245, 254, 256
Golgi, C., 158–9, 170
Golgi cells, 208–10
gonads, 106
gorillas, 55
granular cells, 208–10
'greed sleep', 147
Grossman, S. P., 125
group therapy, 141
growth hormone, 240
guarana liana, 132
Gudden, B. v., 77

hallucinations, hallucinogens, 133,
   136, 139–40, 181–3, 201, 218–9,
   238
hamsters, 254
Han, W., 197
Hannover, A., 154
hashish, 121, 129–32, 145–6
Hassler, R., 108
heart-lung machine, 14, 19
Heath, R. G., 99, 118
Hebb, D., 218–20, 222
hedgehogs, 54
Heimann, H., 87–8, 90–1
Helmholtz, H. v., 163
hemp, 129, 132, 146
hens, 100
Herodotus, 28
Herophilos, 29–30
heroin, 121, 130, 133–5, 140,
   145–51, 239–40
Hess, W. R., 95–7, 108, 114, 232
Hindus, 129
hippocampus, 110–11, 257
Hippocrates, 28
Hitzig, E., 65, 69, 83–4
Hodgkin, A. L., 163, 169
Hoebel, B., 126–7
Hoffmann, A., 139
Hoffmann drops, 144
Holst, E. v., 100
'holy mushrooms', 130, 182
Homo erectus, 55

homunculus, 70
hormonal glands, 34, 104, 106
hormones, 106
horses, 70, 112
Hudgins, C. V., 189
Huxley, A. F., 163, 169
Hydén, H., 251, 253, 260
5-hydroxytryptophan, 235
hypophysis (pituitary gland), 34
hypothalamus, 34, 102, 104–6,
    112, 125–7, 232

immunity barrier, 22
Incas, 130
input, 204, 207–8
insects, 195
insect-eaters, 54, 112
insulin, 125
interpretative cortex, 79
ions, ion pump, 166–8, 172

Jacobsen, A., 253–4
Jacobsen, C., 86
Janzen, R., 69
jelly-fish, 52
Jones, E., 136
Jouvet, M., 233–6, 238
Jovanović, U. J., 226, 230–1

Katz, B., 163, 176
Kety, S., 121, 196
'killer' rats, 126–7
King, M., 126–7
Kito, K., 19
Kleist, K., 69
Kleitman, N., 228–9
knee-joint reflex, 187
Koestler, A., 112, 121, 215

Laird, C., 197
Lashley, K. S., 38, 249, 253
laughter, 109
learning, 10, 40, 46–7, 196, 241,
    246–7, 249, 252–63
Leary, T., 139
leeches, 195
Leeuwenhoek, A. v., 153

Leineweber, B., 24–5
lemurs, 55
Lenin, 66
leucotomies, 45, 87–93
librium, 143, 240
Lilly, J. C., 57
Lima, A., 86–7
limbic system, 102, 109–10, 112,
    115, 125, 257
lithium, 179
Löbsack, T., 12
Locke, John, 259
locus coeruleus, 233–4, 236
Loewi, O., 163
Long, C., 144
LSD, 121, 131, 139–40, 145, 182
Luria, A. R., 78, 92–3

macaque, 56
MacLean, P., 111
Magoun, H., 103
mammals, 54, 111–2, 194, 231,
    238
manias, 110, 131
Mao Tse-tung, 216
Marcus Aurelius, 31
marihuana, 129, 146
mast tree, 132
Matussek, N., 180
Maupassant, Guy de, 144
McConnell, J., 244, 252–3, 262
McCulloch, W. S., 38
medulla oblongata, 34
memory, 10, 83, 108–11, 196,
    244–63
memory, long- and short-term,
    246–8, 254
memory substances, transmission,
    244–5, 252–7
meninges, 35
meprobamate (Miltown), 143
mescalin, 140, 145, 182
methylatropine, 127
mice, 56–7, 126–7, 197, 199, 245,
    255, 261
mid-brain, 34, 54, 232
Miller, H., 149

Milner, P., 97–8
Miltown, 143
Miner, N., 192
mitochondria, 155–6, 171–2
molecular layer, 207, 210
moles, 54
Molière, 177
monkeys, 13–6, 21–2, 45, 47–8,
　55, 70, 94, 99–100, 112, 116–9,
　202, 250
monoaminoxydase (MAO), 179,
　181
morphine, 131, 133–5, 140, 145,
　147, 150
Moruzzi, G., 103, 232
mossy fibres, 207–10
mother love, 124
motor cortex, 68–72, 76, 79, 81,
　83–5, 93, 206–7
muscarin, 182
mussels, 53
myelin, 156, 170
Myers, R., 38–40

narcolepsy, 99
narcotics, 137, 239, 241
nerve fibres, 91, 153–60, 163–4,
　167, 169–74, 184–6, 188, 192–5,
　201, 207–10
nerve gap, 171–2
neurone theory, 158–60
Newman, E. A., 242–3
Niemann, A., 135
nightshade, 133, 145
noradrenalin, 125, 175, 178–82,
　234–6
normal sleep, 230–1, 233–4, 240
nucleic acids, 250–1
nutmeg, 143

occipital lobe, 61, 71–2, 93
occupational therapy, 141
octopus, 53
Olds, J., 97–9
olfactory bulb, 32
opium, 132, 134, 150, 177
opossum, 56

optic chiasma, 39, 45
optic nerves, 39, 193–4, 201–2
Orwell, G., 114
Oswald, I., 239–42
output, 204, 207–8
oxytocin, 106

"pacifist" rats, 126–7
pallium index, 57
parallel fibres, 208–10
parietal lobe, 61, 93
Parr, W., 256
Pavlov, I. P., 89, 189
Penfield, W., 59–61, 73–4, 76,
　79–81
peptides, 255–60, 262
peyote (cactus), 133, 140, 182
phenacetin, 136
phenothiazines, 240
phrenology, 62–3
pia mater, 35
pigs, 70
pituitary gland, 34–5, 102, 106
Plato, 29, 31
pleasure centres, 97–100, 103, 110,
　118–9, 121
pneuma psychicon, 32
polyps, 52
Portmann, A., 56–7
potassium, 166–8, 172–3, 179
potentials, electric, 164–8, 171–3
primates, 54–5
progesterone, 124
prohibition, 150
proteins, 156, 251, 254–5
psychoactive drugs, 89, 129–52,
　177–8, 180–1, 196, 235, 239,
　241, 261, 265
psychosomatic illnesses, 143,
　265
psychosurgery, 85–93
psychotherapy, 141, 261, 265
Ptolemy I, King, 29–30
Purkinje, J. E., 154, 207–9
Purkinje cells, 207–10
puromycin, 254
pyramidon, 136

rabbits, 56, 231, 251
rage, 95–6, 105, 110, 117–8, 219
Ramon y Cajal, S., 158–9
Raphé system, 233–4, 236
rapid eye movements (REM),
  REM sleep, 228–34
rats, 97–9, 123–5, 191, 231, 245,
  249, 251, 253–6, 261
reflexes, 186–91
regeneration, 192–4, 252
repletion (satiation) centres, 99,
  125
reserpine, 181, 234–5
resting potential, 164–8, 172, 175
reticular formation, activation
  system, 103–4, 232
retina, 39, 72, 185, 193–4, 251
ribonucleic acids (RNA), 251–4,
  257–9, 262
ribosomes, 156
Rig-Veda, 129
Robinson, B. W., 120
Rolandic fissure, 69–71
Ropp, R. S. de, 147
Rosenblith, W., 8
Rothschuh, K., 32–3

Saint Paul, U., 100
Schafer, C. R., 114
Scheibel, A. B. and M. E., 103
Scheidt, J. v., 147
schizophrenia, 89, 118, 131, 139,
  144, 181–2, 196, 240
Schlote, W., 211
Schmidbauer, W., 182–3
Schwann, T., 154
scotophobin, 255–7, 260–1
sea-snails, 195
Semon, R., 248
sensory cortex, 71–2, 79, 81
sensory deprivation, 212–3,
  218–24
serotonin, 175, 178–9, 181–2,
  234–6
Sertürner, F., 134
sexuality, 109–10, 123–4
Shebalin, V., 78

Sherrington, C., 163, 225
show trials (Moscow), 215
shrews, 54, 112
Sidman, R., 199
skull, fractured, 27
sleep, 225–43
sleep centres, 231–4
sleep deprivation, 235–40
sleep, stages of, 231, 238–41
sleeping tablets, 131, 136–9, 144
sleepwalking, 229
Smirnov, V., 108
Smith, D., 126–7
Socrates, 259
sodium, 19, 166–8, 172–3, 179
Soemmering, S. T. v., 154
Soma, 129, 133
sparrows, 56
speech centres, 64–5, 73–80, 83,
  85
Sperry, R. W., 40–1, 50, 191–4,
  196
spinal cord, 13, 53, 101, 158, 187,
  190–1, 234
spirit theory, 31–3, 36
split brains, 37–50
sponges, 52
squid, 168–70, 172
star cells, 208–10
stegosaurus, 54
stimulus threshold, 173
storage vesicles, 171–2, 181
Stoyva, J., 241
Suda, I., 19
Suedfeld, P., 223
suicidal tendencies, 142
synapses, 170–9, 184, 186, 198,
  202, 234

tadpoles, 192–3
tea, 131–2, 138–9, 146
temperature eye, 104
temporal lobe, 61, 81, 93
terminal bouton, 171–4, 179
testosterone, 123–5
tetanus toxin, 175
thalamus, 34, 102, 104, 106–9,

112, 232
thalidomide, 137
thyroid gland hormones, 106,
  240–1
tobacco, 130–1, 145, 148–9
tranquillisers, 131, 143–4, 239
transmitter substances, 172,
  178–83
Treviranus, G. R., 154
Tritonia (sea-snail), 195
tryptophan, 178–9
tyrosine, 178

Ungar, G., 255–7, 260–1

valium, 143
vasopressin, 106
Vernon, J., 212–3, 220–4
veronal, 137
vertebrates, 53–4
Vesalius, 33
visual cortex, 71–3, 76, 79, 81,
  83–4, 93
Vogt, C. and O., 68

Volta, A., 162

Wada, J. A., 48
Waldeyer, W., 158
Walter, W. G., 201
Watson, G., 133
Water metabolism, 104, 148
Wedge, B., 218
Welcker, H., 63
Wernicke, C., 74, 76
whales, 56–7
White, R. J., 13–25, 202
Whitteridge, D., 185
Willows, A. O. D., 195–6
Winterstein, H., 227
wiring diagram, 185
withdrawal symptoms, 147–8
Wolin, L., 15
'wrong connections', 190–4, 201

Young, J. Z., 7

Zippel, H. P., 256